Human Nutrition

Fourth Edition

Mary E. Barasi,

BA, BSc, MSc, MRSH
Senior Lecturer in Nutrition,
South Glamorgan Institute of Higher Education, Cardiff

R.F. Mottram,

MB, MS, MBc, PhD
Senior Lecturer in Physiology,
University College, Cardiff

Edward Arnold

© Mary E. Barasi and R.F. Mottram 1987

First published 1948
Edward Arnold (Publishers) Ltd, 41 Bedford Square, London WC1B 3DQ

Edward Arnold (Australia) Pty Ltd, 80 Waverley Road, Caulfield East, Victoria 3135, Australia

Edward Arnold, 3 East Read Street, Baltimore, Maryland 21202, USA

Reprinted 1951, 1954 (with amendments), 1957, 1960
Second edition 1963
Reprinted in paperback with amendments 1972
Reprinted 1974, 1976
Third edition 1979
Reprinted 1981, 1982, 1985
Fourth edition 1987

British Library Cataloguing in Publication Data

Mottram, R.F.
   Human nutrition.——4th ed.
   1. Nutrition
   I. Title   II. Barasi, Mary E.
   613.2   TX353

   ISBN 0–7131–4554–4

Text set in 10/11 pt Plantin Compugraphic
by Colset Private Ltd, Singapore
Made and printed in Great Britain
by Richard Clay plc, Bungay, Suffolk.

Preface

Food is a fundamental necessity for life. All living organisms must provide themselves with sufficient amounts of various substances, termed nutrients, to maintain themselves and perform normal activities.

Knowledge of the nutrients needed by man, and their functions, forms the basis of the science of nutrition. This is essentially a 20th century science, with new discoveries still being made. Although initially a very academic subject, largely the province of chemists and physiologists, nutrition has matured into a broad-based subject, drawing from many disciplines.

Nutrition can no longer be viewed as a study only of the nutrients and their role in the body. The modern definition of the science of nutrition is that of the study of the whole relationship of man with his food. This includes those aspects involved in the supply and procurement of food as well as the way in which deficiencies or excesses consumed can lead to disease. This is obviously far wider in its scope than the mere study of the nutrients.

Nutritional topics now appear regularly in the media and many people are interested in the subject. This is coupled with the general growth in interest in health and an awareness of preventive medicine. Terms like 'cholesterol', 'fibre' and 'vitamins' have become part of everyday language. This is not really surprising, we all eat and so everyone has something to say in discussion on the subject. As food and nutrition are inseparable, many people, as consumers of food, consider themselves 'experts' on nutrition.

Due to the continued increasing awareness of nutrition, accurate information and advice is vital. At best, confusion follows from misinformation, at worst harm can result.

What people eat has far-reaching consequences. Firstly, there is considerable evidence from data on morbidity and mortality of the influence of diet upon health. These influences probably begin in childhood, so the early introduction of healthy eating is important. Accurate education is necessary from a young age.

Secondly, our food choices determine food production patterns, both in our own countries, and globally. Again the consequences of these can be extensive, and damaging. The 1980s have seen severe food shortages in many parts of the Third World, with major famines in several African countries. Even where famine does not occur, foods are in short supply. Part of the blame lies with the West, with its demand for plant foods which are either grown on the better lands in the Third World, or animal foods, which are reared often on feedstuff grown in Third World countries. In both cases, food for the indigenous populations of these countries has to be grown on remaining, often poor quality land, sometimes with disastrous consequences.

Thirdly, the demand for food increases pressures on the producers and manufacturers to produce increasing amounts, and ever-different consumables.

Sometimes this involves the use of production techniques which the public may find objectionable, such as intensive rearing of animals, or the use of large numbers of additives of various types. Public concern about the long-term effects of additives is growing and there is a slow trend away from their use.

Thus the conflict between the desire for adequate supplies of healthy, nutritious food and the consequences of its production is as yet unresolved. It is worth remembering this dilemma in considering the practical aspects of nutrition.

The recognition of the importance of nutrition for health is only gradually gaining ground. In 1983, the National Advisory Committee on Nutrition Education (NACNE), and in 1984, the Committee on Medical Aspects of Food Policy (COMA) published documents outlining changes that should be made to the British diet in the future. They also pointed the way to radically new ways of thinking about nutrition.

The time therefore is right for a new edition of this book. There is a need for the fresh approach pioneered by the NACNE Report to become widely disseminated, so that all can benefit from this new approach to eating for health. The more flexible approach to food, looking at the overall diet, and moving away from the concepts of basic food groups is a feature of this new edition.

Several areas of the book have been expanded since the third edition. These include aspects of nutrition which have increased in importance, or where further advances in knowledge have occurred. The study of dietary fibre and its role in prevention of disease is included. Another aspect concerns fat, how much should be eaten, whether this should be of plant or animal origin and its overall involvement with health. The social aspects of nutrition have increased in importance in the last decade, with the recognition that social situations and pressures may be the major determinants of the ability to obtain a healthy diet. This part of the book has therefore been expanded, to take into account such groups as the elderly and the ethnic minority groups, both of which are increasing in number in Britain. There has been an upsurge of interest in sport and fitness; the needs of sportsmen are thus also considered. Finally, a small but growing number of the population are turning to alcohol or other drugs; these also have implications for their nutritional intakes.

Chapters on food hygiene and food processing are no longer included in this edition. The effects of food processing on specific nutrients have however, been briefly included in the respective chapters. Readers wishing a more comprehensive treatment of the subject are referred to texts on food science. Although food-borne disease still occurs, perhaps more frequently than before with the increased use of deepfrozen food and microwave cooking, its direct importance to the nutritionist has perhaps become less. The food microbiologist and the community physician are the members of the public health professions who are more directly concerned.

Throughout the text, the male personal pronoun has generally been used, for simplicity; this does not of course imply any bias against the female, and is merely used for clarity.

The book is intended as an introductory text in all aspects of the subject of human nutrition; this includes the roles of nutrients, their provision in food, as well as the 'human' side – the needs and social pressures on the consumers of that food.

The text offers a fresh approach to nutrition, adopting the recommendations proposed by NACNE in 1983. We hope the book will provide a starting point for those who wish to study the subject in greater depth, in the more specialized textbook in various branches of nutrition. For those whose study allows no opportunities to pursue the subject further, it remains a broad and scientific foundation in nutrition.

While one of the two authors of this new edition (RFM) is the son of the late Professor V.H. Mottram (the first author of this book), and a medically qualified physiologist, the other (MEB), studied Physiology at Chelsea College, London, and later, Nutrition at the (then) Queen Elizabeth College in London, where VHM was the first professor.

Our approach to the subject is determined firstly by a consideration of the needs of the human body for various nutrients, if it is to carry out its normal functions and avoid different disease states. Secondly, we appreciate that everyone is individual in their approach to nutrition, so our considerations are tempered by the social constraints on people as individuals. It is with these two themes in mind that we have prepared this book.

1987   MEB
                                                                               RFM

Acknowledgements

The authors wish to acknowledge the permission of the Controller of Her Majesty's Stationery Office for the use of data from *The Composition of Foods, the Household Food Consumption and Expenditure Survey, Recommended Daily Amounts of Food Energy and Nutrients for Groups of People in the United Kingdom (Report 15)* and *Diet and Cardiovascular Disease (Report 28)*. They would also like to thank Dr J.S. Garrow for permission to reproduce Figs. 3.2, 3.4 and 3.5 from his book *Treat Obesity Seriously*.

The considerable help of Mr John Robertson with word processing is also gratefully acknowledged.

Contents

1

People and Food: The Science of Nutrition

Nutrition is about food and the people who eat it. Frequently studies of nutrition leave out this second aspect – that of the actual consumer of the food – and concentrate on the chemical aspects. Such accounts may focus on the constituents of the food, the nutrients, what happens to them within the human body and what the results are if insufficient amounts are provided. But the individual is also important. It is all very well to talk about isolated nutrients; however people do not eat 'nutrients' as such, but food. In choosing what food to eat, a great number of factors influence the choice. For different people, the relative importance of these factors will differ, depending on their cultural backgrounds and the varying circumstances of their lives, such as money, cooking facilities and knowledge. This subject is explored further in Chapter 12.

Few of us are that 'average' person who appears in nutritional statistics, in figures for recommended intakes or in the National Food Survey results. It is important to bear this in mind whenever we meet average figures, and consider how our individual situations make us different from the 'average' person.

Nutrition is defined here as the study of the relationship between people and their food. This chapter briefly considers these two aspects: people and the food they eat. The question of why people eat, and what nutrients they obtain from their food, is discussed. The methods that nutritionists use to acquire further information about nutrition are also considered.

Why do we eat?

Physiological needs

This may seem to be a fairly obvious question, and the initial reaction may be to answer 'because of hunger', or even 'to keep alive'. Both of these points are true: the body has a physiological need for food, and when deprived for a short period of time, various reactions produce sensations of hunger.

A brief explanation of physiological need may be necessary. Physiology is the study of the way living organisms function. These functions will only proceed normally if the environment inside and outside the body's cells is controlled within fairly narrow limits. Maintaining this constant environment requires the input of energy and nutrients, which can be summed up in the term 'physiological needs'.

If we are deprived of food for long periods of time, then the body has to draw on its reserves so that weight is lost. Ultimately, if food is not provided (but water is available) the withdrawal of protein from the reserves reaches such a level that death may occur from heart failure, following protein depletion of the heart's muscle. However, in a previously well-fed individual this may take as much as 60 days; it is hardly fair to claim that every meal is preventing death from starvation!

In the Third World countries many people do eat largely because they are hungry – they may be hungry most of the time – and the threat of starvation from lack of food is very real. However, in the West, and in a country such as the United Kingdom where food supply is plentiful and regular, our food intake is generally ruled by stimuli other than outright hunger, or the fear of starvation.

Habit

In the West, food is available at just about all hours of the day or night. People do not, however, eat continuously, but usually at fairly clearly defined 'meal times', with 'snack times' interspersed between them.

Eating has therefore become a habit. We eat because it is the time to do so, and often because someone has prepared a meal. A survey performed by the British Nutrition Foundation in 1984 on adults and children aged 11 to 15 years, found that the majority of these had at least six 'eating occasions' per day. These included several 'non-meals' (their description for snacks), which were described as occasions when one type of food only was taken, and included drinks such as tea or coffee, as well as biscuits, chocolate or sandwiches. Seventy-two per cent of adults had four or more such 'non-meals' in a day. In addition, 48% of adults had one 'meal' per day, which was described as a selection of different separate items, eaten with a knife and a fork and usually requiring time to prepare, cook and eat. The eating of 'meals' (as opposed to 'non-meals') was generally thought by the respondents as being important for health. The survey also showed that 65% of respondents ate something between 11:45 a.m. and 2:45 p.m., with 71% of people having their main meal in the evening during the week. On Sunday, however, a meal in the middle of the day forms the main meal in 63% of households. On Saturday, half have their main meal in the middle of the day, and half in the evening.

The need for fairly organized mealtimes in a society run according to the clock can be appreciated. Chaos would ensue, if in every office, classroom and business organization people wandered off to eat when they felt like it! A degree of organization is essential, both from the consumers' and the cooks' point of view. It may be argued that this rigorous timing of meals is introduced too early in life. There is still a tendency to feed infants in their first months of life according to the clock, usually four-hourly. The more relaxed approach of 'on demand' feeding gives the infant the opportunity to be fed when it is actually hungry. It does, however, introduce a considerable measure of uncertainty into the mother's life, as she cannot always predict when the baby will require feeding.

Some people may eat just because food is available. They are unable to resist the desire to eat and are apparently less sensitive to their own internal cues about needing food. Being unable to leave, or waste, food may cause problems with some mothers of young children. If the child always leaves food on its plate, the mother tends to finish it up and so she overeats, since this food is additional to her own intake.

Psychological influences

Apart from these external drives to eat, there are also internal influences. Boredom provides a major incentive to eating – it fills many empty hours for some people. Depression may also make people turn to food for comfort; the food may provide emotional security. This stems from the reassurance given by food provided by parents to children. It is important that the 'food as comfort' response is not made too frequently, as it is likely to result in overweight – with its own associated emotional problems! These may then set up a cyclical pattern of behaviour which is very difficult to break. For some people, eating becomes compulsive, and the consequences of overeating, feelings of fullness or gain in weight, may result in such behaviour as self-induced vomiting or the taking of excessive amounts of laxatives. This has been termed 'bulimia nervosa'; people (usually women) with this problem need help to re-establish a normal eating pattern, and explore the reasons for the disturbance.

Sensory appeal

Certain aspects of the food itself also increase the drive to eat. These include its sensory appeal – how it stimulates the senses, initially by its appearance and smell, later by its taste. In the British Nutrition Foundation survey, mentioned earlier, the taste of food was of prime importance, and the majority of people admitted to eating a wide variety of favourite foods. Among adolescents, a key feature was also the apearance of the food. The visual appeal of the food, although essential to attract the eye, may be misleading in its message. In addition, nutritional judgements are made on the basis of appearance. For example, white eggs have largely disappeared from sale in the United Kingdom, but in the USA they are preferred to brown eggs. As the (unfounded) 'superiority' of brown eggs has been accepted by UK consumers, so people no longer want to buy white eggs, and vice versa in the United States.

A wide variety of foods offers encouragement to eat. Studies on both animals and people have shown clearly that when offered a variety of food, total intake was greater than when just a single food was offered. Thus it is possible to make rats overweight by offering them a 'cafeteria diet', containing chips, hamburgers, crisps, chocolate, etc.; with ordinary rat pellets, they simply do not eat enough. It also explains how people, having eaten apparently to their fill of a main course, can still manage to eat something sweet afterwards. Overweight is much less common in communities around the world where only a few foods regularly appear in the diet – it seems that monotony imposes its own limits on eating. On the other hand, organizing food into different courses, with different flavours, seems to enhance food intake.

Social influences on eating

As well as providing personal pleasure, food may also be used in a social context to please (or displease) others. Food may be used by a small child as a tool to manipulate its parents. The child may refuse to eat to express feelings of anger, jealousy, insecurity, to gain attention and to exert control over its parents. They unwittingly reinforce this behaviour by becoming concerned about the child's eating, offering different foods and generally making a fuss.

Foods which are disliked may be eaten to please the provider of the food – maybe a parent, friend or partner. Visitors to another country may be put in this position by their hosts and find themselves obliged to eat foods which are alien and possibly unappetizing to them, or risk offending their hosts.

All of these influences and some of their interrelationships are summarized in Fig. 1.1. The factors influencing food habits and food choice are further discussed in Chapter 12.

The nutrients in food

After eating, food is digested by the enzymes of the gastrointestinal tract and broken down to release its basic constituents – the nutrients. This will be true regardless of the type of food eaten, unless it is completely indigestible.

What happens to the food?

When food is eaten the physical chewing and grinding action of the teeth, the mixing and churning in the stomach and the mixing in the intestines help to break the pieces of food down into smaller fragments. The mixing also brings the fragments into close physical contact with the various secretions of the digestive tract

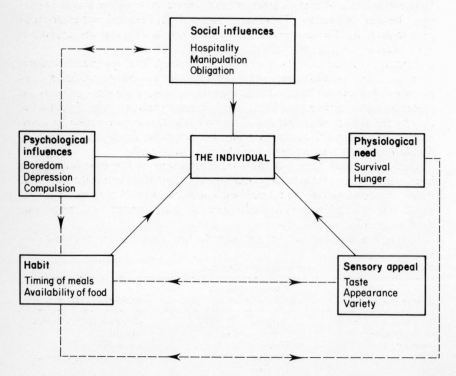

Fig. 1.1 Why do we eat?

which break down the chemical bonds, changing the nutrients into simpler chemical substances which the body can absorb from the intestines.

Not all of the food that is eaten can be fully absorbed, despite the fact that the process of digestion is extremely efficient. Fat and protein are almost completely digested and absorbed. In a healthy person about 3 to 4 g of fat appear in the faeces per day; this comes mainly from the bacteria in the large intestine. Similarly, the 10 to 20 g of protein in the faeces come principally from bacteria and disintegrated cells which lined the digestive tract.

It is the complex carbohydrates in food, like cellulose and the hemicelluloses together with lignin, which escape the digestive enzymes. Traditional thinking considered these carbohydrates as useless to the body, calling them 'roughage' and considering them as irritants to the bowel. It is now known that they are partially fermented by the large-bowel bacteria, which use them as an energy source for their own needs. The portion that actually appears in faeces is quite altered from the form found in food. Although the products from the complex carbohydrates are largely excreted from the body, their presence in the large intestine serves an important role in the health of the intestines, and possibly other parts of the body. They are therefore an essential part of the diet, and only 'indigestible' as far as the body's own enzymes are concerned. The digestion of the major nutrients is considered in more detail in Chapters 4 to 6.

What are the functions of the nutrients?

Whatever mixture of foods is eaten, its basic constituents will be simple or complex chemical substances. These serve essential physiological and biochemical roles in the body. The nutrients are introduced here briefly; they are looked at in more detail in subsequent chapters.

Nutrients can be classified in various ways. The traditional approach has been to look at their predominant roles in the body: energy-providing nutrients – carbohydrates and fats; building and repairing nutrients – proteins and some minerals; regulating nutrients – some minerals and vitamins. However this may be misleading, since many of them have several roles and cannot be conveniently slotted into one particular group. An alternative functional classification (Table 1.1) shows that nutrients fulfil several possible roles.

Another approach is to divide nutrients according to the amounts needed by the body. Those required in relatively large amounts (tens of grams) are the *macro* nutrients – proteins, carbohydrates and fats. These contrast with nutrients needed in small amounts (a few grams, milligrams or micrograms) – the *micro* nutrients – the minerals and vitamins.

This type of division does not prejudge the role of nutrients in the body.

Table 1.1 Functional classification of nutrients

Energy provision	Tissue formation/ maintenance	Regulation of functions
Fats	Proteins	Complex carbohydrates
Carbohydrates	Carbohydrates	Vitamins
Proteins	Fats	Minerals
	Minerals	Proteins (as hormones)
	Vitamins	

Carbohydrates

These are the main group of nutrients in our diet. They may be simple or complex carbohydrates; this distinction is important when considering their functions in the body. The simple carbohydrates (commonly called the sugars) primarily supply energy, providing 16 kilojoules per gram, and very little besides this. They also form part of some of the structural components of the body: in cells, the nervous system and in joints.

The complex carbohydrates (starch and glycogen) also supply energy; they are associated with other nutrients, especially minerals and vitamins, and also some protein. They are thus more nutritionally valuable than the simple carbohydrates. In addition, some of the indigestible complex carbohydrates (cellulose, hemicelluloses) help to maintain the health of the intestines and probably reduce disease in many other systems of the body.

Fats

Dietary fats are primarily seen as concentrated sources of energy, supplying as they do 37 kilojoules per gram of fat. In addition to the major group of dietary fats, which are triglycerides, the diet also contains quantities of cholesterol and a small amount of phospholipid. These play a part in other functions in the body, concerned mainly with cell membrane structure. Thus they cannot be regarded solely as energy-providing. In addition there has been considerable interest in the last twenty years concerning the types of fatty acids comprising the triglycerides, with a suggested link between these and the occurrence of coronary heart disease.

Associated with the fats are the essential fatty acids, which are converted to substances in the body known as prostaglandins and their derivatives. These play a variety of roles, including a regulatory function in blood platelet aggregation (and thus in blood clotting) and in cell membrane structure and function.

Proteins

These are chains of amino acids which are obtained from food and then reassembled into proteins typical of the body. A certain number of amino acids can be converted into new ones, not present in the ingested food. However, this facility does not extend to all the amino acids; some, called 'essential amino acids', must be supplied in the food as needed. These are then used to build or repair body tissue, make good the losses occurring from normal body metabolism and for other essential synthetic processes in the body. Any amino acids which are present in amounts surplus to requirements are broken down and part of their structure is used to supply energy. Energy obtained from proteins in the living body is equal to 17 kilojoules per gram. Thus as well as providing the basic materials from which the cells, enzymes, nervous system transmitters and some hormones are made, some protein is used to provide energy. This last function is in fact a wasteful fate for the most expensive component of our diet.

Vitamins

These are an assorted group of organic substances whose common feature is that they are essential in the diet for the health and well-being of man. The corollary of this is that when any are absent, a deficiency disease may develop, related to the particular vitamin which is lacking.

Vitamins are commonly divided into water-soluble and fat-soluble subgroups. The water-soluble group contains all of the B complex and vitamin C. Some are relatively unstable on cooking and all are easily lost from the body in regular daily amounts.

The fat-soluble vitamins, vitamins A, D, E and K, are generally found in association with fat-containing foods. They are absorbed when normal fat absorption takes place in the intestines, and they are generally stored in the body, usually in the liver or adipose tissue. Excessive amounts of vitamins A and D can be harmful; no harmful effects from excessive vitamin E or K have been reported. These fat-soluble vitamins are more stable on the whole than the water-soluble group, so are less easily destroyed in foods.

The various vitamins have a wide variety of actions in the body. These include carbohydrate, fat and protein metabolism and regulation; cell division and differentiation; formation of all tissues and blood; stabilization of membranes; and formation of blood clotting factors. It can be seen that the vitamins are a diverse group with many varied functions, which are considered in more detail in Chapter 8.

Minerals

The body contains a large number of inorganic elements, some of which have probably entered as contaminants and do not therefore have a recognized physiological or biochemical role. They may in fact hinder some of the normal metabolic processes. The majority do have identifiable functions and in their absence, clinical deficiencies may occur. The most prevalent mineral is *calcium*: an adult man may have 1.2 kg of it in his body, and it is an essential component of the skeleton, helping to maintain hardness and rigidity. The calcium in the skeleton also acts as a reserve for the blood calcium. A small amount of calcium is found in the plasma and contributes to the blood clotting pathway. It also regulates the activity of muscles and nerves. In addition to calcium, the bones also contain *phosphorus* in slightly smaller quantities than calcium.

Sodium and *potassium* are present in the blood and tissue fluids. Together, these control the distribution of fluid in the body between the extracellular and intracellular compartments. They are also responsible for the small electrical charges on cell membranes, needed for nerve impulses and muscle contraction. Although these electrolytes derive from the diet, their levels are regulated principally by hormones within the body.

Iron, of which there is only some 6 grams in the body, is an essential constituent of the oxygen-carrying pigments, haemoglobin and myoglobin. Inadequate levels of iron result in low levels of these pigments, and consequently a poor supply of oxygen to the tissues. This is iron-deficiency anaemia, which results in tiredness, weakness, pallor and breathlessness. The red blood cells are paler and smaller than normal.

Zinc, present in similar quantities to iron, is an essential component of a large number of enzymes in the body, as well as being needed for protein synthesis. A deficiency of zinc results in growth failure and poor wound healing as a result of the failure of protein synthesis to proceed normally.

There are many other minerals found in the body, which include copper, cobalt, selenium, magnesium, chromium, fluoride and iodine. They have diverse roles, but in general they act as cofactors for enzymes, or form a key part of some other substance found in the body. In most people eating their normal diet, it is unlikely that a deficiency of one of the less prevalent minerals would occur. However, if the diet becomes abnormal, contains few foods or a large amount of just one food, or when there is extra stress on the body, such as following injury or illness, or when rapid growth occurs, then the chances of deficiency increase.

Sources of nutritional information

Present knowledge about nutrients, their deficiencies and the effects of these on health has come from a variety of sources and a number of different techniques. To assess the effect of diet on health, information both about the diet and the state of health of a population is needed. Neither of these is easy to obtain. The available information usually originates from whole populations, rather than individuals. This means that a particular finding about the relationship between diet and health may be true when considering the population as a whole, but may not apply to any one particular person in that population. The exceptions to the general trend are usually identified by those who want to question the existence of the relationship. Exceptions inevitably exist – there is no such person as the 'average man'.

A further problem inherent in attempting to establish the relationship between diet and health is the finding that there are very few situations in which the diet is the only contributory factor causing health or ill-health. One exception might be a clear-cut nutritional iron deficiency anaemia, caused by a shortage of dietary iron. Even here, some women may be anaemic due to the combined effects of poor dietary iron intake and perhaps heavy menstrual losses of iron. Thus in the majority of diet-related disorders, diet is only one of several contributory factors. Its actual importance in the development of the disease may be very difficult to assess. This is particularly true of the diseases that currently receive a great deal of attention because of their prevalence in the West. These include obesity, high blood pressure, coronary heart disease and cancer of the colon.

Population studies

General surveillance

In the United Kingdom, information pertaining to nutritional status is obtained routinely from continuous studies which provide very general surveillance on health and food intake. At present these include:

(1) Consumption level estimates (MAFF)
(2) Household Food Consumption and Expenditure Survey (MAFF)
(3) Birth and mortality statistics (OPCS)
(4) Hospital inpatient enquiry (DHSS)
(5) Hospital activity analysis (district health authorities)
(6) Blood transfusion returns (DHSS)

Note:
MAFF = Ministry of Agriculture, Fisheries and Food
OPCS = Office of Population Censuses and Surveys
DHSS = Department of Health and Social Security

Consumption level estimates provide information on the total amount of food available to the country from all sources. Many countries draw up such estimates which provide a very general picture only of food availability within a country.

The *Household Food Consumption and Expenditure Survey* provides a continuous report of the food coming into households for consumption. It does not take into account food bought and eaten outside the home, nor does it consider food distribution within the home. It also provides information about the amount of money spent on food by households of various composition, economic grouping and in different geographical locations within the country.

Birth and mortality statistics are indicators of the general health of the nation, and nutrition obviously plays an important role. For example, the health of women before and during pregnancy may determine its outcome. So perinatal mortality statistics may be a reflection of the health of women. These figures showed a dramatic fall during the Second World War in Britain from 38 per 1000 to 28 per 1000, this during a period when pregnant women received priority rations. More recently, supplementation of the diet of undernourished women in some parts of the world has reduced perinatal mortality.

Records of the causes of death provide indicators of the incidence of particular diseases and may allow correlations with particular dietary patterns to be tested. Thus coronary heart disease deaths show a significant positive correlation with fat intakes in many countries of the world.

Hospital statistics – obtained from the DHSS on hospital admissions – provide information about the incidence of disease, both regionally and nationally. Recent trends in the incidence of rickets and osteomalacia in the United Kingdom have been followed using these data. The Blood Transfusion Service monitors the status of the blood offered by volunteers and this also allows the trends in anaemia among this population to be monitored. In the years between 1954 and 1980, this had fallen from 8% to 4% among females donating blood. It must be remembered that these figures may not be typical of the general population. In fact there is evidence that iron deficiency anaemia is again increasing in Britain in the 1980s.

Statistics such as these from hospitals require a well-organized health service which collects, records and stores the information. This may not be available in many countries as a method for nutritional surveillance.

Epidemiology

The information obtained from such national surveillance may be considered in relation to that from other countries with similar – or different – disease patterns. Inspection of the data may demonstrate correlations between particular aspects of diet and certain diseases.

It is on the basis of work such as this that the differences between countries in the incidence of coronary heart disease and different fat intakes were found to be correlated (see Fig. 1.2). Similarly the incidence of hypertension in different countries has been shown to be correlated with the intake of salt. Work in Africa showed that

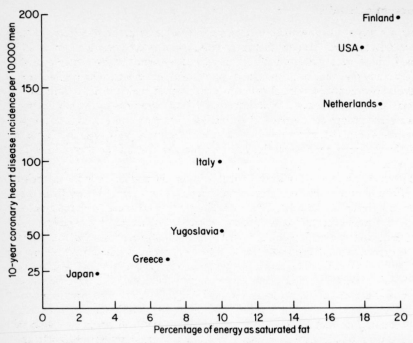

Fig. 1.2 Relationship between the percentage of dietary energy provided by saturated fats and the 10-year coronary heart disease incidence per 10 000 men, initially aged 40–59 years (based on Keys Seven Country Study, 1970).

many bowel disorders seen in the West were unknown there, and this is probably linked to the considerably higher intakes of dietary fibre consumed in some of these countries compared with the relatively low levels eaten in the West. These types of studies are known as epidemiological, that is they look at different patterns of disease in large population groups. Studies of this nature point to a possible link between two factors (the disease and a particular pattern of eating) which could be related in that population. One major shortcoming of this approach is that the relationship may not necessarily apply to any one particular person. This could be because the genetic make-up or behaviour reduces susceptibility to the nutritional factors causing the disease. These exceptions will always occur, but if our population sample is large enough, then the overall trend will be sufficiently clear to demonstrate the relationship in the population as a whole.

Studies of groups of migrants are particularly useful. Often a specific group of people has moved (for a variety of reasons) to another country, where the environment may be very different. Sometimes new patterns of disease emerge in this situation, which were unknown in the country of origin. Thus it seems that adoption of the customs of the host country may result in disease, or reduce the risk of a disease which occurs in the parent country. A study of the customs which have been adopted may be a valuable guide to those factors which contribute to these diseases. This approach has been used for example, in the study of Japanese migrants to Hawaii, or Jews migrating to Israel. It may be a valuable key to the understanding of rickets and osteomalacia among the migrants of Asian origin settled in the United Kingdom.

Intervention studies

Some scientists are unwilling to take such studies as proof of a relationship between factors, and demand that intervention studies are performed on populations. In these, the study group of the sample undergo some change; in the case of a dietary study they may be given a food supplement, or advice to change their diet. There is also a control group, matched in every respect, which is left to continue its normal life style. After a period of time, usually as long as possible, any differences between the groups are assessed. It is then assumed that if any change in disease pattern has occurred, and if the only change in the study group was that brought about by the study, then it was this change which had caused the alteration in disease pattern.

In practice, however, it is fairly difficult to alter just one aspect of the diet without affecting others. For example, asking people to eat more dietary fibre may result in a greater intake of fat, if the extra fibre is taken as bread (with more butter on it), as breakfast cereal (with milk and sugar), or as jacket potatoes (filled with butter). Asking people to reduce their salt intake may also cause a reduction in total energy intake, as many processed foods – often high in fat, sugar and salt – may be excluded from the diet. The reduced energy intake may cause weight loss, and so reduce blood pressure, which is one of the changes that is expected following a salt reduction. In addition, the normal life style followed by the control group may also change with time, so that the baseline for comparison is different.

Information on dietary intake and individual nutritional status may also be obtained from smaller groups. Usually this may be carried out on people who are suspected of being nutritionally at risk, such as young children, pregnant women or the elderly. Several such surveys have been performed in the United Kingdom in recent years by the Department of Health and Social Security or bodies such as the Medical Research Council. They have identified nutrients which may be in short supply and provided evidence of nutritional deficiencies among members of such groups.

Dietary intake studies

Information on dietary intake is usually obtained by weighed inventory or food records. The 'diet history' is used by dietitians in hospital or community work.

(1) *Weighed inventory*. In this method all the food eaten by the subject during a period of one week is weighed and recorded, together with any plate waste. Actual nutrient intakes are then calculated using tables of food composition values, such as those of McCance and Widdowson which are widely used in the United Kingdom. (Other countries have tables giving analytical data for foods common in their own countries, and local tables should be used where possible.) This technique, when carried out over a seven-day period, gives a reasonably good estimate of dietary intakes. It is, however, very dependent on the cooperation of the subject, and because many people may find it tedious, low levels of cooperation may result. However, with support and help from the research workers, it is a successful technique.

(2) *Food records*. This is a technique in which the food eaten is simply recorded in a notebook by the subject, without being weighed. Some attempt may be made to

quantify the food, either in terms of household measures (e.g. spoonsful or cupsful), or by accurate and detailed description of the food (e.g. 2 egg-sized boiled new potatoes). The information obtained in this way is less precise than that provided by weighing, but the reduced constraint on the subject does increase the level of cooperation. This method may provide a sufficient level of accuracy for the needs of the study. For example, if the study aims to identify those within the population studied who have high, medium and low intakes of a particular nutrient, this information can be supplied adequately by descriptive techniques only.

A technique developed in 1984 uses a photographic method for recording the food eaten. The subject is supplied with a camera and photographs the food he is about to eat, from a set distance. The food is also described in a notebook. The slides produced from these photographs can then be compared with a library of slides showing preweighed food samples, so that quantities may be assessed. The technique can give acceptable results in the hands of a skilled researcher. The novelty of the technique and its ease of use make it an attractive method for subjects and therefore may increase cooperation.

(3) *Diet interview*. A technique which is widely used to obtain a general picture of a person's food intake is the interview. In the hands of a skilled dietitian this can elicit an accurate picture of a person's dietary habits – the diet history. This will be sufficient to pinpoint potential excesses or deficiencies. The interview may be more or less detailed, depending on the sort of information required. It usually consists of general questions about the daily eating pattern, along the lines of 'What do you usually have for breakfast, mid-morning, lunch, etc.'. It then aims to draw a more precise picture by focussing on the current (or previous) day's intake, by asking 'What did you have for breakfast, mid-morning, lunch, etc. today or yesterday?'.

Most people are so unaware of what they eat that it is often quite difficult to remember even the previous day's food. For this reason, a diet interview usually asks about the food eaten only over the previous 24 (or at most 48) hours. The dietitian may also try to obtain some idea of food portion sizes – often with the use of food models, showing sizes of typical servings. A checklist of foods may also be used to remind the subjects about foods that they do eat, but forgot to mention.

The diet interview, or diet history, is valuable as a means of obtaining a picture of someone's general eating. Its main limitations are:

(a)   It depends on people actually having a pattern of eating. Some people eat so haphazardly that a pattern does not exist and so 'usual intake' cannot be established.

(b)   It is dependent on an awareness of what is eaten. This awareness does not exist in children up to 13 or 14 years old. It may also be fading in an elderly person. Also, it is generally greater among women than men, so that an interview with some men may uncover areas of vagueness about food intake.

(c)   It depends on the accuracy of the subject's memory. Even the most well-motivated subject may simply not remember everything they have eaten.

None of the methods so far described give a precise and absolute measure of nutrient intake. This lack of precision is generally acceptable in survey work. However, there are occasions when a greater degree of accuracy is needed. The technique used is the preparation of duplicate meals, one of which is eaten by the subject, the other analysed for its nutrient content. It is only in this way that really accurate figures will be obtained. Obviously this sort of approach is impossible and unnecessary for household survey work, and generally only takes place in hospital metabolic wards.

Assessing nutritional status

To complement the data concerning food intake, some other assessment of nutritional status may be required. This can be obtained by clinical examination, anthropometry, or biochemical (or biophysical) tests. One or more of these methods may be used concurrently to present as complete a picture of the nutritional state of the person as is necessary for the purpose of the study.

(1) *Clinical examination*. This involves looking at the body and detecting changes in its external appearance. Quite a number of nutritional deficiencies may cause alterations in superficial structures. A clinical examination may include the hair, face, eyes, mouth, tongue, teeth, gums, glands (such as the thyroid), skin and nails, subcutaneous tissue (to detect fat thickness, oedema) and the musculoskeletal system (to note bone deformities, muscle wasting). Some internal organs like the liver may be felt, and reflex tests may be performed to test nerve pathways and muscle function. A trained observer will be able to detect many of these changes, which may be very confusing to an untrained eye. Even then, results from clinical tests are usually supplemented by other tests.

(2) *Anthropometry* literally means 'measuring man'. Various measurements can be made; by relating these to standards typical of the test population, deviations may indicate abnormal nutritional status. Included here are weight and height measurements. In children, these are related to standard growth curves. These may be used to indicate the rate of physical development of the child, especially when sequential readings are taken over a period of time. Figure 1.3 shows a growth curve for recording weight in boys aged 2 to 10 years.

Curves are also available for recording other parameters, such as height, head size, etc., and for different age groups. Measuring head and chest circumference gives an indication of relative growth of the brain and body and in children is a useful index of protein-energy malnutrition. In well-nourished infants, the chest circumference becomes greater than that of the head from 6 months, but in protein-energy malnutrition this does not occur.

Arm circumferences coupled with skinfold thickness measurements give a measure of muscle development (or degree of wasting). Skinfold measurements at midbiceps, midtriceps, subscapular and suprailiac sites are used as a measure of the amount of fat in the body. The technique of skinfold measurement is shown in Fig. 1.4.

(3) *Biochemical measurements* (or biophysical). These require a sample of tissue or body fluid from the subject. The commonest samples used are blood and urine, although analysis may also be performed on samples of hair or bone marrow. Actual blood levels of particular nutrients may be measured, and expressed in relation to the expected normal value. In addition, the activities of various enzymes which either depend on a specific nutrient, or reflect the body's level of a nutrient, may be assayed. Using urine samples, the baseline level of excretion of a nutrient may be measured. This will reflect recent intake. For nutrients which are not

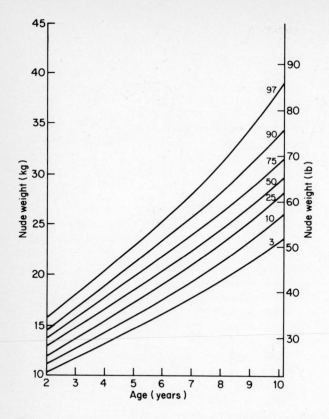

Fig. 1.3 Standard growth curves for boys aged 2–10 years (nude weight).

stored in the body, a 'loading' dose may be given and a repeat measurement made in the urine to detect the amounts retained by the body.

Bone marrow biopsies will show the blood-forming cells; calcium stores in the bone can also be measured by bone biopsy. X-ray examination of the bone can detect stage of bone development or rarefaction in ageing. Finally it is possible to measure the levels of some trace elements in the hair, although the scientific accuracy of these assays is not proven.

Measurement of the body's metabolic rate uses the whole body as its sample tissue. These measurements may be performed on subjects where there is a suspicion of abnormally high or low metabolic rates. The equipment used can be very elaborate (whole body calorimeters) or relatively simple (oxygen-consumption measuring appliances). For details of these techniques, see Chapter 3.

Using such equipment, a considerable amount has recently been learned about the differences in metabolism between people and the influence of food on metabolism.

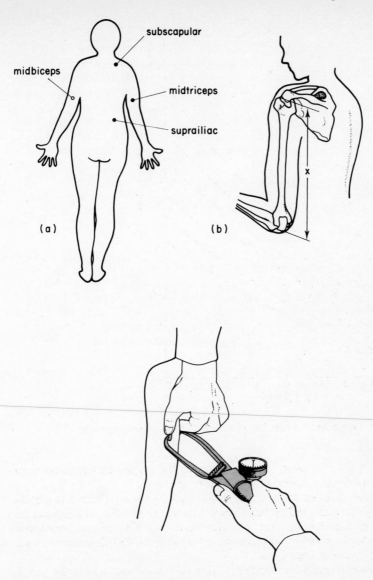

Fig. 1.4 Measurement of skinfold for assessment of body fat content. **(a)** The four commonest sites used for measurement are subscapular, suprailiac, midbiceps (note that the open circle indicates front of upper arm) and midtriceps. Measurements from all four sites are added together for use in formulae to obtain body density and hence fat mass. **(b)** For midtriceps measurement, the midpoint of the upper arm is found. **(c)** The Harpenden calipers are shown in use. The skinfold measures a double layer of skin and sub-cutaneous fat. A lengthwise skinfold is firmly grasped between thumb and forefinger, avoiding underlying muscle. The calipers are applied about 1 cm below the operator's fingers, and the fold is held gently throughout the measurement. Three measurements are made and the results averaged.

Feeding trials

These represent a somewhat different approach to the question of nutritional assessment. They have a long history, and are still a valid means of examining (and improving) nutritional status. A nutritionally at-risk group (for example, poor, pregnant women) is given a nutritional supplement. A carefully matched group is maintained on their normal diet. The trial may continue for a period of months or even several years (spanning a number of pregnancies in the example used here). At the end of the feeding period any differences noted in the supplemented group compared with the unsupplemented controls will be attributable to the supplement. This depends on good initial selection of the two groups, to ensure comparability; this may be quite difficult to achieve.

Feeding trials on high-risk groups provide valuable evidence on nutritional status as well as directly evaluating the effects of a supplement.

Nutritional knowledge has grown considerably in the last twenty years, yet there is still much to learn. Perhaps it is true to say that as many questions have been raised as answered. The information has come from large-scale epidemiological studies which have pointed the way for prospective studies. It has also come from many smaller studies which have highlighted problems in specific groups, using nutritional assessments and dietary surveys. Finally, clinical nutrition, working within the hospital setting, has often worked empirically with the sick patient, discovering special nutritional needs and how to meet them. Observation and intervention have come together in the treatment of such nutritional problems and have broadened our knowledge in this area.

2

Essentials of Practical Nutrition

This chapter looks at how foods may be combined to achieve what might be considered a healthy diet. As seen in Chapter 1, people eat for a variety of reasons; one of these reasons may be to achieve health. This is a factor of importance for many people, as can be seen from the recent growth in the health-food industry in the United Kingdom. In 1985 a major British supermarket chain introduced a series of 'healthy eating' leaflets on subjects such as fat, protein, fibre, salt, vitamins and minerals and fitness. These leaflets were intended to complement major nutritional labelling, which was also introduced. Public interest in this has been extensive and other supermarket chains are now following this example.

The belief that nutrition can promote good health is not new, but the nature of the argument has changed recently. This follows the publication of the NACNE report in 1983. The report is a 'discussion paper on proposals for nutritional guidelines for health education in Britain'. The traditional view of a diet compatible with health has been that of a 'balanced' diet.

The balanced diet

This concept is based on the idea that if sufficient amounts of various nutrients are present, then health will ensue. The amounts deemed to be sufficient were usually those which were not associated with signs of malnutrition, or nutritional deficiency. Thus the idea of a balanced diet was that of a mixture of foods which prevented nutritional deficiency and therefore, by implication, resulted in health. Nutritional information made available to people was based on this idea and, as such, was appropriate. However, this information may become inappropriate with the passage of time, yet it has become ingrained as part of the 'received wisdom' of the nation, and may be difficult to change. Any novel ideas may be seen as confusing, unless the reasons behind them are examined.

For example, after the First World War vitamins were being discovered, and there was considerable interest in the way that these (together with the minerals in our food) could protect against some of the nutritional deficiencies then found. One of these, rickets, affected large numbers of children, especially in the urban areas. Vitamin D and calcium were the nutrients which protected against rickets. Milk is a good source of both of these nutrients; it therefore earned a reputation as a 'good food for children'. This idea has persisted, although for the majority of the British population rickets is no longer a threat. This reduction in the incidence of rickets has come about for a variety of reasons. These include the use of fortified margarine, the availability of vitamin drops for children and the reduction in atmospheric pollution.

Another nutrient commonly believed to be essential in large amounts for children is protein. Growth does involve the laying down of protein in the body, so the need for dietary protein seems obvious under these circumstances. In the days when many children were generally underfed, a shortage of protein and other nutrients did indeed result in poorer growth and small stature. Now, people in the West eat perhaps too much protein, yet the ingrained belief persists that milk, eggs, cheese, meat and fish – all sources of animal protein – are essential for the growth of children. But children who are vegetarian, or even vegan (eating no animal protein foods at all), have been shown to grow perfectly well and be developmentally comparable to meat-eaters. We are now also aware that the sources of animal protein listed above are particularly high in fat, and particularly the saturated fats. The fat component may contribute to an excessively high total fat intake, which is considered harmful to health. In addition, the saturated fatty acids may be associated with a higher risk of heart disease. For these reasons, animal protein foods are generally considered less nutritionally desirable than they once were. To change the prevailing attitude about their central role in growth however, requires a fundamental re-education.

A great number of similar misconceptions surround the carbohydrate-containing foods. In many people's minds they are seen as providing essential energy for work ('a Mars a day helps you work, rest and play'), yet also as being particularly fattening (mainly bread and potatoes). The confusion arises from the fact that the various carbohydrate sources are not distinguished from one another, so that all are seen as energy providers only, with their additional nutritional benefits being disregarded. The belief that bread and potatoes are fattening derives from, and was probably reinforced by, reducing diets which required that these foods be restricted or eliminated from the diet. What was never explained was that any 'fattening' property arises from the fats that are generally eaten together with these foods, rather than from the bread or potatoes themselves. Advertising campaigns that have tried to educate people about the nutritional value of bread have resulted in only a brief halt in the downward trend of bread consumption. The general belief that bread is fattening is still widespread. Similarly, the poor reputation of the potato also persists.

Sugar products, which are correctly perceived as providing energy, are additionally believed to possess other beneficial properties; the belief that sugar is necessary in the diet is prevalent. This is completely unfounded, since the glucose to which the sugar is ultimately changed is obtainable directly from other carbohydrates in our food. Glucose is also made from proteins when the need arises. From the biochemical point of view, sugar has no essential role in the diet as a source of glucose for the body. Since sugar provides no other nutrients, it is truly nonessential from every viewpoint. On the other hand, there may be some occasions when a readily absorbed dose of sugar is useful, such as for diabetics or athletes. For the majority, glucose can be obtained in a much more useful form, with many other nutrients, from the complex carbohydrates in our diet, such as starch, rather than from sugar.

There is another misconception about nutrition which seems to have grown in parallel with the growth of the slimming industry. This is the idea that some foods are 'fattening', while others are 'slimming'. This seems to have its roots in many weight-reducing diets, in which certain foods – the 'fattening' ones – are prohibited, while others – the 'slimming' ones – are encouraged. This makes little nutritional sense: all foods provide the body with energy. It is of course true that weight for weight, some foods are higher in energy than others. Consuming 8.4 MJ in the form of supposedly 'slimming' foods will have the same effect as 8.4 MJ provided by supposedly 'fattening' foods. In other words, the actual food has no inbuilt property to cause weight gain or weight loss. What counts is the amount of it which is eaten.

These common nutritional beliefs are being based on ideas which were appropriate in their time. They are also mainly concerned with achieving 'balance', thus preventing deficiency due to a lack of one or more specific nutrients. This concept of health is one of absence of disease, and thus somewhat negative.

The healthful diet

It may be argued that the aim of preventing nutritional deficiency has largely been met in our western society. Nutritional deficiencies caused primarily by a lack of appropriate food intake are now relatively rare. When it does occur, nutritional deficiency may be precipitated by other factors, such as physical or mental disease, or the cultural and dietary habits of particular population groups. However, low income, ignorance or adverse social conditions may still result in inadequate nutritional intakes and be the cause of deficiency. There is nevertheless a growing awareness that nutrition is not simply a question of preventing nutritional deficiency, and that good nutrition can have a positive role to play in promoting good health.

Mortality statistics in western countries show that we are far from 'healthy'. Conditions such as coronary heart disease, stroke and cancers result in 581 860 deaths (or 61% of total mortality) in England and Wales each year. Epidemiological data suggest that diet has a role to play in these conditions. By modifying our diets and choosing foods which are 'healthier', better health is likely to follow. The NACNE report suggested that the diet to aim for should no longer be called a 'balanced' diet, with all of its connotations of preventing malnutrition. In its place, the 'healthful' diet is proposed. This is a diet aiming to promote positive, better health for the whole population, rather than the negative avoidance of deficiency by the vulnerable few.

If there were certain foods available that contained all the nutrients required, then eating a diet for health would simply involve eating sufficient amounts of these foods. It might be rather monotonous, but we could be sure of meeting our nutritional needs. The only such food, however, is human milk; even this only satisfies all the nutritional needs of the infant up to about six months of age. Thereafter, other foods must be added to the diet, to maintain its nutritional adequacy for the growing infant. For the rest of our lifespan a mixture of foods must be eaten to satisfy nutrient needs.

Staple foods

For most of the peoples of the world, the basic diet is straightforward and made up of just one or two foods, which are termed 'staples'. These are generally cereals (wheat, rice, maize, millets) or starchy roots and tubers (potatoes, cassava, yams and taro). To add interest to the staple foods and to introduce variety, the diets contain various meats, fish, vegetables, fruits and spices. The greater the availability of these additional foods, the less is the emphasis placed on the role of the staple food in the diet. This is the pattern seen in western countries, such as the United Kingdom; but even here the staples – wheat and potatoes – appear in various forms at practically every meal.

People who have migrated to the United Kingdom may bring their traditional dietary patterns with them, so that other combinations of 'staple plus variety' are seen. For example, rice will be eaten by Bangladeshis, some people from India as well as Chinese immigrants from Hong Kong, Malaysia and Vietnam; West Indians may eat starchy roots as their staple food. Wheat remains the staple amongst people from eastern and southern Europe and some parts of India and Pakistan. Having a staple food does not mean that other cereals or roots are not eaten; they simply comprise a smaller part of the diet.

As the staple food is such a central feature of the diet, it must provide a significant number of nutrients. This is indeed so, especially in the case of cereals. They provide not only significant amounts of energy, but also protein, B vitamins and some minerals. Wheat is the cereal with the greatest nutritional quality, with maize, millet and rice providing smaller amounts of nutrients. In general, the staple roots have a lower nutritional quality than the cereals, particularly the roots eaten in some of the tropical countries; the analysis of some cereals and roots is shown in Table 2.1.

The concept of building meals on the basis of 'staple food plus variety' reflects the primary need for energy and protein in the diet; these are supplied by the staple food. The 'variety' components of the meal come from a selection of different foods, and supply minerals, vitamins and some additional protein and energy.

In addition to providing energy, protein and additional nutrients, the staple food also should contain some dietary fibre, the amount depending on the degree to which the cereal has been processed or refined. In their natural, whole state, cereals and roots contain quite large amounts of dietary fibre. Fibre in the diet has the benefit of providing satiety, or a feeling of repletion after eating. A good staple food as the cornerstone of the diet thus provides both energy and satiety. However, if a staple food is processed and refined, it is quite likely to lose its major satiety-providing component, namely the dietary fibre. As a result, the energy provided by the staple has a correspondingly smaller satiety effect. There are two possible, related consequences: firstly, feelings of hunger may persist after a normal intake of energy. Secondly, and as a result of this, additional food may be eaten to achieve satiety, with a consequent overconsumption of energy and gain in weight.

Not all of the satiety obtained from a meal comes from the staple food, but as an important item in the diet it has a major contribution to make to the satiety. A diet is unlikely to consist exclusively of staple; all cultures diversify their staple foods with items to add variety of tastes, flavours and textures.

Foods to add variety

These foods may be present in relatively small quantities and yet contribute significantly to the nutrient intake. Foods in this group include animal products – meats, dairy products and eggs – as well as various plant products – fruit, vegetables, herbs and spices. The variety of dishes in which these can be presented

Table 2.1 Nutrient contents of some staple cereals and roots (per 100 g). N indicates that the analysis has not been done directly; it should not be assigned the value zero; a value from a similar or related food should be used. From: Paul, A., Southgate, D.A.T. (1978), McCance and Widdowson's *The Composition of Foods*, and Tan, S.P., Wenlock, R.W., Buss, D.H. (1985) *Immigrant Foods* (Second Supplement). London: HMSO.

	Energy (kJ)	Protein (g)	Dietary fibre (g)	Fat (g)	CHO (g)	Calcium (mg)	Iron (mg)	B_1 (mg)	B_2 (mg)	Nic.a. (mg)
Wheat flour										
wholemeal (100%)	1351	13.2	9.6	2.0	65.8	35	4.0	0.46	0.08	5.6
white, plain (72%)	1493	9.8	3.4	1.2	74.8	140	2.2	0.31	0.03	2.0
Rice (polished, raw)	1536	6.5	2.4	1.0	86.8	4	0.5	0.08	0.03	3.0
Oatmeal (raw)	1698	12.4	7.0	8.7	72.8	55	4.1	0.50	0.10	1.0
Rye flour (100%)	1428	8.2	N	2.0	75.9	32	2.7	0.40	0.22	1.0
Millet flour	1481	5.8	N	1.7	75.4	40	N	0.68	0.19	2.8
Maize grits (raw)	1515	8.7	N	0.8	77.7	4	1.0	0.13	0.04	1.2
Cassave (fermented, dried – gari)	1469	1.0	N	0.8	77.7	45	1.6	0.08	0.03	1.0
Plantain (raw)	379	1.2	2.2	N	22.4	5	0.2	0.03	0.02	0.4
Taro tuber (raw)	393	2.2	N	0.4	20.2	34	1.2	0.12	0.04	1.4

CHO = carbohydrate; Nic.a. = nicotinic acid.

is almost endless. However they are prepared and eaten, they will contribute valuable nutrients to the diet. The greater the variety eaten of these additional foods, the greater the likelihood that an appropriate mixture of nutrients is obtained.

On the other hand, a diet that contains very little variety may be lacking in some essential nutrients. In addition, a diet that contains a great proportion of refined and processed foods may also be at risk of causing nutritional deficiency. In this case, the consumption of a variety of foods may *not* protect against deficiency. The reasons for this can be explained using the concept of *nutrient density*.

Nutrient density

All foods supply energy. However the actual amount of energy in 100 grams of different foods is very variable. Most foods also contain some nutrients; again, the actual amount of any nutrient present per 100 grams of the food will vary considerably between different foods. One way of comparing the nutritional value of different foods is to look at their relative contents of a particular nutrient, expressed per 100 grams of food. For example:

Bread (white): 991 kJ and 100 mg calcium per 100 g
Milk: 272 kJ and 120 mg calcium per 100 g
Boiled potatoes: 343 kJ and 4 mg calcium per 100 g

Of these three foods, milk provides the most calcium on a weight-for-weight basis, and potatoes the least. Bread is the richest source of energy of the three.

An alternative way of comparing these foods, which takes into account the energy they supply, is to calculate how much nutrient (calcium in this particular example) they contain per 1000 kilojoules of the food. The nutrient content is then expressed in terms of 1000 kilojoules of energy supplied by the food. In this example we find that:

White bread supplies 101 mg calcium per 1000 kJ
Milk supplies 441 mg calcium per 1000 kJ
Boiled potatoes supply 12 mg calcium per 1000 kJ

This means that if a person ate enough of any one of these foods to provide 1000 kJ, they would also obtain the amounts of calcium listed. The concept of density (density = mass/volume) can be used to describe the amount of the nutrient present in relation to a unit of energy (1000 kJ in this case). On this basis, it can be concluded that for the foods above, milk has the highest 'calcium density', bread the next and potatoes the lowest. This provides us with a useful means of comparing different foods in terms of the nutrients they provide per unit of energy. It is possible to perform similar calculations on all foods, to show their relative nutrient densities, for all the nutrients they contain. Some foods may have very low densities for particular nutrients.

Two extreme examples of foods which have zero nutrient densities for all nutrients are refined, white sugar, and spirits (such as gin, vodka or whisky). Both of these dietary items supply only energy, with no accompanying nutrients. They are sometimes called 'empty energy', as they are devoid of all other nutrients.

The meals in Table 2.2 show that for most nutrients the density is higher in meal 2 than meal 1, indicating the greater nutritional value of meal 2. The exceptions are carbohydrate, fat and vitamin D. The higher carbohydrate density derives

Table 2.2 The use of nutrient density calculations to compare the nutritional values of foods or meals.

	Weight (g)	Energy (kJ)	Dietary fibre (g)	Protein (g)	Carbohydrate (g)	Fat (g)	Calcium (mg)	Iron (mg)	B$_1$ (mg)	Vit. C (mg)	Vit. D (μg)
Meal 1											
Tomato soup	150	345	0	1.2	8.9	4.9	25.6	0.6	0.04	0	0
White toast	50	633	1.4	4.8	32.5	0.9	55.0	1.1	0.08	0	0
Margarine	20	600	0	0	0	16.2	0.8	0.1	0	0	1.6
Mars bar	60	1112	0	3.1	39.9	11.3	96.0	0.7	0.03	0	0
Coca Cola	200	336	0	0	21.0	0	8.0	0	0	0	0
Totals		3026	1.4	9.1	102.3	33.3	185.4	2.5	0.15	0	1.6
Meal 2											
Baked potato	150	546	3.0	3.1	30.5	0.2	12.0	0.9	0.12	12.0	0
Cheddar cheese	50	841	0	13.0	0	16.7	400.0	0.2	0.02	0	0.13
Baked beans	150	405	10.9	7.6	15.5	0.8	67.5	2.1	0.10	0	0
Tomato	50	30	0.8	0.4	1.4	0	6.5	0.2	0.03	10.0	0
Fruit yoghurt	140	567	0	6.7	25.1	1.4	224.0	0.3	0.07	2.5	0
Milk, whole	225	612	0	7.4	10.6	8.6	270.0	0.1	0.09	3.4	0.06
Totals		3001	14.7	38.2	83.1	27.7	980.0	3.8	0.43	27.9	0.19
Meal 1 Nutrient density (amount of nutrient/1000 kJ)			0.5	3.0	33.8	11.0	61.2	0.8	0.05	0	0.5
Meal 2 Nutrient density			4.9	12.7	27.5	9.2	327	1.3	0.1	9.3	0.06

from the Mars Bar and the Coca-Cola, both of which are high in sugar but low in the other nutrients. They therefore 'dilute' the nutrients present in the remaining part of the meal. The fat density is a little higher in meal 1, because of the use of margarine. The margarine, fortified with vitamins, also contributes to the greater vitamin D density of meal 1.

Many refined and processed foods tend to have low nutrient densities. This may arise for one or both of the following reasons.

(1) Nutrients which were originally present in the whole food may be removed during refining; this occurs in the milling of wheat where the outer layers, rich in minerals and vitamins, are removed and discarded. The remaining flour has a disproportionately high level of energy-providing starch, and relatively lower levels of other nutrients.

(2) The processing of foods often includes the addition of fats and sugar. As a result the energy content of the processed food is increased. Therefore any nutrients present in the food will have lower densities because of the raised energy content.

It follows that if the diet contains a large proportion of such foods, with distorted nutrient densities, the resulting energy intake may be quite high (possibly excessively high), but the nutrient levels may be far too low. In the extreme situation where a large amount of sugar or alcohol is consumed, the energy from these may account for perhaps half of the day's total energy need. As this energy has no accompanying nutrients, all the necessary nutrients have to be met from the remainder of the day's intake. Unless this comprises foods with high nutrient densities, nutritional deficiency may well result. If the remainder of the diet contains predominantly refined or processed food, then some nutrients are likely to be in short supply. Overt signs of nutritional deficiency may not actually appear, but there may be a reduced state of well-being and possibly an increased susceptibility to illness. This is likely to be most serious in those groups that have special nutritional needs, as a result of growth or other physiological stresses.

This is not just a remote possibility. Detailed studies of the typical diet eaten by the British population, using MAFF data, show that in 1985 the average diet provided enough energy and protein, excess sodium, chlorine and phosphorus, and was short of a very extensive list of other nutrients, including starches, fibre and essential fats with their associated vitamins D and E. Vitamin B_6, folic acid, biotin and the minerals potassium, magnesium, iron, zinc, copper, selenium and chromium may also have been in short supply.

Constructing a diet

A summary of the principles outlined in this chapter can serve as the foundation for assembling a daily diet. A suggested scheme is given in Fig. 2.1.

Most of the world's diets, and certainly the ones represented by various ethnic groups in the United Kingdom as well as those of the indigenous population, will fit into this basic scheme. It may be argued that some of the British population plan their meals by starting from the animal foods (stage 2) and adding the staple (stage 1) and vegetables (3) later. However, the choice of the staple is in fact so fundamental that its selection is automatic – we do not even need to say that, for example, there is toast for breakfast, or potatoes as part of the evening meal. Bread

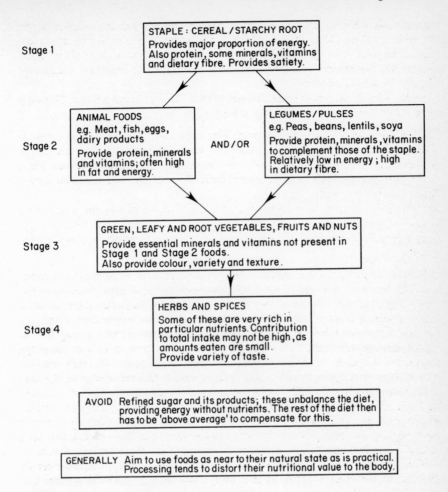

Stage 1

STAPLE : CEREAL / STARCHY ROOT
Provides major proportion of energy.
Also protein, some minerals, vitamins
and dietary fibre. Provides satiety.

Stage 2

ANIMAL FOODS
e.g. Meat, fish, eggs,
dairy products
Provide protein, minerals
and vitamins; often high
in fat and energy.

AND / OR

LEGUMES / PULSES
e.g. Peas, beans, lentils, soya
Provide protein, minerals, vitamins
to complement those of the staple.
Relatively low in energy ; high
in dietary fibre.

Stage 3

GREEN, LEAFY AND ROOT VEGETABLES, FRUITS AND NUTS
Provide essential minerals and vitamins not present in
Stage 1 and Stage 2 foods.
Also provide colour, variety and texture.

Stage 4

HERBS AND SPICES
Some of these are very rich in
particular nutrients. Contribution
to total intake may not be high, as
amounts eaten are small.
Provide variety of taste.

AVOID Refined sugar and its products; these unbalance the diet,
providing energy without nutrients. The rest of the diet then
has to be 'above average' to compensate for this.

GENERALLY Aim to use foods as near to their natural state as is practical.
Processing tends to distort their nutritional value to the body.

Fig. 2.1 Constructing a diet.

and potatoes are already assumed to be 'on the menu'. The planning process has
therefore started with the staple, but it is often not made explicit, with the result
that the first conscious stage becomes stage 2 (or stage 3 in the case of vegetarian
diets). Thus it would seem that even in the United Kingdom this planning scheme
does apply.

The actual amounts of these foods to be eaten is considered in Chapter 11.

3
Energy in Nutrition

Until 1900 the energy content of foods dominated the science of nutrition. From then on, as the importance of the qualities of proteins, vitamins and minerals in foods loomed large, their energy content tended to be ignored. This was mistaken. Proper nutrition demands an adequate supply of energy, as well as protein, vitamins and minerals. One without the other three is useless.

From 1939 onwards we began to feel differently, and we now compare the energy-poor diet of poor people with the overabundance of energy of the rich. We are right to worry about energy, for if the energy content of a diet is low due to poverty, we can be sure that proteins, minerals and vitamins will be grossly deficient. Few foods are totally lacking in substances from these three categories, so if the energy content is abundant then some protein, etc. will be absorbed as well. Foods with a high energy content must form the major part of the food we eat. There is no way of doing without the 500 g or so of solid food that must be eaten each day to provide our bodies with their essential energy.

Units of energy

In physics and chemistry the SI unit that is now preferred is the *joule*. The joule was originally defined as the amount of energy expended when a force of 1 newton was exerted through a distance of 1 metre. It was named after Joule, who originally determined the mathematical relationship between heat and physical force. This is now enshrined in the modern use of his name for the basic energy unit. Heat energy used to be defined in separate units, calories. One calorie of heat raised the temperature of 1 ml of water through 1 °C. *This is equal to about 4.18 joules.* Although the joule is now accepted as the basic energy unit in both physics and chemistry, in nutrition the kilocalorie (kcal) – 1000 calories – is still regularly used, so in this book we will refer to both units, since some of our readers are familiar with one and some with the other unit system. The kilocalorie is sometimes written 'Calorie' to distinguish it from the original calorie. Joules, in nutrition, are usually referred to as thousands (kilojoules) or millions (megajoules) of the original units of the physical sciences. Therefore 4.18 kilojoules = 1 kilocalorie.

The reason for this link between physical force, chemical energy of food and heat, is that energy is the one fundamental entity. This is why scientists think of energy in all these forms in the same unit (the joule), whether they are studying the galaxies, the human or simple chemicals. Energy can never (outside atomic nuclear reactions) be created or destroyed, only transformed. It may appear in many forms: the kinetic energy of a speeding bullet or rushing stream, the potential energy of water behind a dam, electricity, light or heat, or physical work. When a man walks upstairs, he does work (measured by his weight, multiplied by the height of the staircase). That work comes from energy liberated by oxidation of food in the body. If he is carried up in a lift, then the electrical energy, itself produced by oxidation of coal in the power station, does the work for him. Both the energy contained in his food and in the coal came from the sun. One could write the following series of energy transformations:

nuclear energy → heat and light → chemical energy in plants → food or coal

food → chemical energy in muscles → mechanical work

coal → heat → electricity → mechanical work

Since energy cannot be lost, only transformed, a definite amount of work must equal a definite amount of heat energy which, in turn, must equal a definite amount of chemical or electrical energy and so on.

It is useful also to remember that the unit of electrical energy consumption, the watt, is also linked to the joule. Something using electrical energy at 1 joule/second is using 1 watt of electricity. The rate of energy use of a typical man, 2600 kilocalories or 11 megajoules of energy each day, is about 100 joules/second or 100 watts. Just feel the heat given off by a 100-watt light bulb and then remember that you are giving off as much yourself.

During a normal day's activity the typical man requires 11 MJ of energy, all of which must come from his food and drink. If the energy content of the food is less than 11 MJ, then he raids the body energy stores (fat). If he eats more than 11 MJ some will be wasted, but some will be added to the energy stores in the fat depots. Each gram of fat contains 37 000 joules (37 kJ) of energy, so our typical man, if he eats nothing for a whole day, can obtain all the energy he needs by using a mere 300 g of his stored fat. He could obtain it by eating this amount of fat. Other foods contain less energy per unit weight and so correspondingly more has to be eaten. We can think of the *energy density* (joules or calories per gram) of foods. Thus to supply 11 MJ of energy a person would have to eat 355 g of butter, 650 g of cheese, 610 to 930 g of meat, 2.75 kg of potatoes, or 11 kg of cabbage or apples. So it does matter from the energy point of view what we eat. Bread, potatoes and vegetables are more bulky and less energy-dense than butter, cheese and meat, so one has to eat more of them; and one's appetite is more readily satisfied with a food intake of lower energy content than if one sticks to the energy-rich butter, cheese and meat.

The measurement of energy

The nutritional scientist has to know both the energy contents of foods that may be eaten, digested, absorbed and then oxidized in the living body, and also the energy production rates of the body when performing various activities. Several methods, direct and indirect, have been devised to obtain these values. We consider first the direct determination of the potential energy of foods eaten by chemical means in the laboratory, and then how we determine the amount of food a person eats. After that we describe how the energy produced by a person from food may be determined. If the physical laws concerning mass and energy conservation apply, we should find that the potential energy of the food eaten equals the energy produced.

The potential chemical energy of foods that can be liberated by complete oxidation is determined by an apparatus known as the bomb calorimeter.

Bomb calorimeter

The word 'calorimeter' is applied to any apparatus that measures heat production, the word deriving from the Latin *calor*, 'heat'. The bomb calorimeter is shown in Fig. 3.1. It is a steel vessel which can be closed with a tight-fitting stopper. It contains a platinum crucible into which a weighed amount of combustible material (pure chemical or food) can be placed. It is filled with pure oxygen under pressure. The food can then be ignited by an electric current, when it will burn explosively. Before ignition the whole is sunk in a stirred water bath, of known volume and temperature, and the food is only fired when the temperature is constant. The heat of combustion is determined from the rise in water temperature, the rate of its subsequent cooling and the specific heat of the calorimeter itself.

Fat and carbohydrate are oxidized to CO_2 and water in a bomb calorimeter, just as in a living body. Fats give about 37 kJ/g, when oxidized in the bomb calorimeter, all the energy appearing at once as heat. In the body, oxidation proceeds in a series of separate chemical reactions; about half the energy is trapped in the 'high-energy compounds' and may then be used for the many other reactions that require an input of energy before they can take place. These include muscular contraction, protein synthesis and growth, gland secretion and the passage of nerve impulses.

In a bomb calorimeter, protein burns to water, CO_2 and oxides of nitrogen or nitric acid. This is highly poisonous, so in the body, protein oxidation stops short of oxidizing the $-NH_2$ groups. These are converted to the harmless and soluble

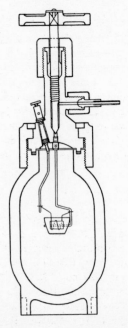

Fig. 3.1   The bomb calorimeter.

compound, urea. (Uric acid is similarly formed as the chief nitrogen-containing remainder of nucleic acids, present in all foods.) The bomb calorimeter can be used to determine the energy content of these substances, normally excreted from the body in urine. The difference between the bomb calorimeter energy value for protein, and the energy value of the urea, etc. derived from the protein, gives the energy available from the oxidation of protein in the living body. This is 17 kJ/g, slightly higher than the figure for starch or glycogen (16 kJ/g).

The reader must be clear that it is the *potential* chemical energy of foods that is being measured in the bomb calorimeter. When we turn from the potential chemical energy of foods to the *actual* amounts of energy liberated by oxidation of these foods in the body, we have to remember both the incomplete oxidation of protein already mentioned, and also that a small proportion of all foods is not fully digested and absorbed from the gut.

In the next section, outlining the way we survey the food eaten to determine energy intakes, we make use of 'food tables', giving energy contents of foods. All these figures are corrected for the potential discrepancies produced by incomplete absorption or oxidation. These corrections have been calculated as a result of extensive, meticulous experimental work and are known as the *proximate principles of energy determinations*. McCance and Widdowson's *The Composition of Foods*, published by HMSO, contains a description of them.

Diet surveys

Knowing the bomb-calorimeter values for foods, it is possible to estimate the energy turnover of a person by determining the energy content of the food he or she eats. Since these methods have been described elsewhere in this book (Chapters 1 and 10) they will not be described here, but we must mention at this point some of the errors and assumptions made in using this way of determining energy intake. These are:

(1) That any food wastage, for instance on utensils or plates, has been weighed and allowed for.
(2) That the person being studied is neither gaining nor losing body weight. This can be checked, but the water content may vary by 1 to 2 litres from day to day.
(3) That the record is an honest, complete and accurate account of food intake.
(4) That the diet recorded is typical of the person's normal intake.
(5) That the conservations of matter and energy are true for the human body.

Human calorimeter

In the human calorimeter, the heat output of a living person is measured directly. This sounds simple in principle, but in practice is a most costly, difficult and boring enterprise. Only a very few human calorimeters have ever been built, the most famous from our point of view being that designed, built and used by Atwater and Benedict in the USA between 1891 and 1903.

In 1976, to enable careful and accurate studies on the body weight changes that follow any imbalance between food energy intake and bodily energy needs, a similar apparatus was built at the British Medical Research Council's Clinical Research Centre near London. In this apparatus were incorporated many new

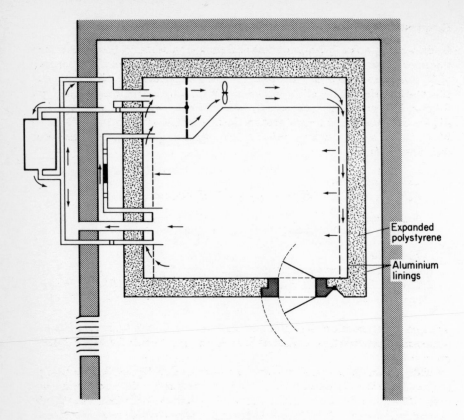

Fig. 3.2 A direct calorimeter. Redrawn from Garrow (1981).

materials and methods of recording not available to Atwater and Benedict 80 years earlier, but the principle remained the same. The construction details ensure that the heat produced by the person living in the calorimeter can be continuously and accurately measured and recorded. A full description of this modern apparatus is given in Dr J. Garrow's book, *Treat Obesity Seriously*. Some of the material in this chapter has been culled from Dr Garrow's book, and we are indebted to him and the book's publishers for permission to reproduce some of his illustrations.

A door and a window allow access to the calorimeter chamber, which contains a bed, chair, table and apparatus for exercise. Fresh oxygen-containing air of the ideal temperature and humidity is supplied by the circuit shown in Fig. 3.2. Food and drink are handed in through the window; urine and faeces are handed out.

While the modern apparatus is less costly to build and run than the original equipment used by Atwater and Benedict, such equipment can only measure a person's energy output in a hospital or scientific laboratory. It could not be used at home, work or in sporting activities. On these occasions, metabolic activity must be measured by some indirect means.

Respiratory quotient

By drawing up properly balanced chemical equations, as shown here, one can see that in oxidation of carbohydrates, the volume of CO_2 produced equals the volume of O_2 consumed. When fat is oxidized however, the volume of CO_2 produced is about 70% of the volume of O_2 consumed. This is usually expressed as a decimal fraction, CO_2 produced/O_2 consumed, called the respiratory quotient (RQ). The RQ for carbohydrates is 1.0 and that for the fat example shown below is 43/60 = 0.717. Other fats have slightly differing RQs, depending on the precise nature of their fatty acids.

Glucose oxidation
$$C_6H_{12}O_6 + 6O_2 \rightarrow 6H_2O + 6CO_2 + 15.5 \text{ kJ/g energy}$$

Starch oxidation
$$(C_6H_{10}O_5)_n + 6nO_2 \rightarrow 5nH_2O + 6nCO_2 + 17 \text{ kJ/g energy}$$

Fat oxidation
e.g. glyceryl butyro-oleostearate (the chief fat of butter)
$$C_3H_5O_3.C_4H_7O.C_{18}H_{33}O.C_{18}H_{35}O + 60O_2 \rightarrow 43CO_2 + 40H_2O + 39 \text{ kJ/g energy}$$

The non-nitrogenous portions of amino acids are, on the whole, intermediate in composition between fats and carbohydrates, and for protein the RQ is usually given as 0.81.

Finally, from these equations, one can emerge with figures for the energy produced in kilojoules for each litre of oxygen consumed in these oxidation reactions. (Those who feel a need to convert these figures to kilocalories should divide the relevant figures by 4.2.) Table 3.1 sets out the values for oxidizing pure chemicals, carbohydrates, fats and proteins, and Table 3.2 extends further the energy production rates and the proportions of fat and carbohydrate oxidizing at different RQs, once the energy production due to protein (the amount of which is calculated from the rate of excretion of urea etc. in the urine) has been determined.

Before concluding this section it must be emphasized that all these relationships are matters of pure chemistry and have all been determined in the laboratory. However, chemical relationships are the same in the living body as in the chemist's apparatus. We can apply the values for energy production from food oxidation that were obtained by chemists nearly a century ago, to studies of human energy needs and production today. This means simply that if one knows either the foods consumed or the respiratory gaseous exchanges, one can calculate the energy transformations in the body. The methods are generally known as *indirect calorimetry*.

Table 3.1 The energy obtained by oxidizing foodstuffs (Zuntz, 1897).

	O_2 needed ml/g	CO_2 produced ml/g	RQ	Energy release kJ/g	Energy released per litre of O_2 used kJ
Starch	830	830	1.0	17.0	21.1
Glucose	747	747	1.0	15.5	20.8
Fat	2020	1430	0.71	39.0	19.6
Protein	966	782	0.81	18.6	19.3

Table 3.2   The energy produced and foodstuffs oxidized at different RQs.

Non-protein RQ	kJ per litre O_2	% Energy derived from Carbohydrate	Fat
0.71	19.6	1	99
0.75	19.8	16	84
0.80	20.1	33	67
0.85	20.3	51	49
0.90	20.6	68	32
0.95	20.8	84	16
1.00	21.1	100	nil

Note that the energy content of foods, determined by the heat energy evolved in the bomb calorimeter, and the heat energy produced when the same foods were oxidized by a living person in the human calorimeter were found by Atwater and Benedict to be the same, to an accuracy of 1 part in 1000. Biological oxidation was proved to be identical with chemical oxidation when the final product (the heat evolved) was measured. We know that the intermediate steps and the speeds of the two reactions are vastly different; but the point was made, once and for all time, that there was no fundamental difference – no 'life force' – involved in the living cell processes, and that the laws of conservation of energy are as true for the living body as for inanimate chemical reactions taking place in a chemist's laboratory.

Respiratory gas measurements

The simplest indirect calorimetric method is that of measuring the rate of O_2 consumption using a recording spirometer. This is simply a gas holder containing oxygen, from which a person can breathe. The expired air is returned to the spirometer, after the carbon dioxide produced has been removed. The volume contained in the spirometer falls, and the rate of fall is recorded and measured, to give the rate of oxygen consumption. It is common practice to assume that each litre of O_2 used causes the production of 20 kJ of heat, so the energy production can be simply calculated.

Until the early 1970s such recording spirometers were becoming increasingly complex and expensive, but now a relatively cheap and simple apparatus has been produced, designed for secondary school use (Fig. 3.3). The main disadvantage of recording spirometers is that it is only possible to study people who are stationary or resting. Furthermore, one can obtain no information about the foodstuffs being oxidized, since measurements of CO_2 production and calculation of RQ are not made. The method depends also on the subject breathing regularly, i.e. inhaling equal volumes at regular intervals. A sigh or cough, even swallowing saliva, can disturb the record for as long as a minute. Most recording spirometers must be refilled after 10 to 15 minutes.

Early this century, another method for the collection, measuring and analysis of expired air was developed by Haldane and Douglas at Oxford. Large rubberized canvas bags, holding 75 to 150 litres, were used to collect the air. After a measured period of time the air in the bags was mixed, a sample taken for analysis, and the volume determined. Bags could be carried on their backs by people employed in various activities, though the bulk of a 150-litre bag interferes considerably with activities such as cutting or loading coal at a mine's coalface.

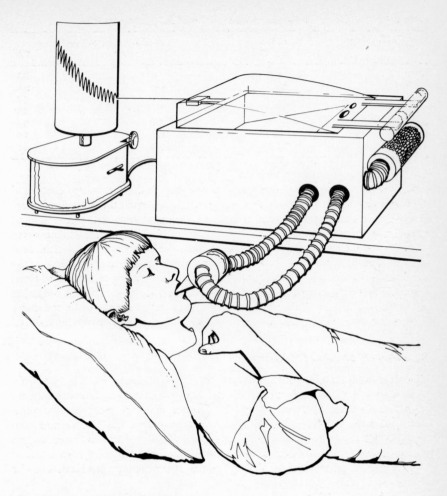

Fig. 3.3 The recording spirometer.

In the 1940s and 1950s two devices were developed which have partly replaced the bag technique. The Kofranyi-Michaelis respirometer is a small mechanically driven gas meter and sampling device which measures the volume of the expired air and takes a proportion of the air into a sample container for subsequent analysis. The Integrating Motor Pneumotachograph (IMP) does the same, but volume measurement and sample collection are performed electrically. The whole apparatus is smaller and lighter than the K-M machine.

Another technique, using a ventilated hood through which air is blown continuously and which fits comfortably over a recumbent subject's head, was developed in the 1970s. This depends upon the accurate analysis of the very small changes in oxygen and carbon dioxide produced when the subject adds the relatively small amount of expired air to the larger ventilating airstream flowing through the hood.

It is a method that causes minimal disturbance to the subject. Like the spirometer, however, the hood can only be used with a stationary and recumbent subject.

Most of these techniques require a chemical or physical analysis of the samples of expired air, which is usually performed at some time after the samples are collected. The development of a simple means of gas analysis and the miniaturization of electrical equipment has enabled the design and production of the Oxylog. This not only measures expired air volumes and takes proportional samples, but it also determines the difference in oxygen concentration between the samples and atmospheric air. An electrical circuit then calculates and displays the oxygen consumption automatically from these measurements. The whole apparatus weighs 2.5 kg and fits into a small leather carrying case. The subject wears a fitted mask over mouth and nose, as in the K-M and IMP machines, which is connected to the apparatus with a flexible corrugated tube. The Oxylog was designed at the MRC's Clinical Research Centre and described to the Physiological Society in 1977, by S.J.E. Humphreys and H.S. Woolf (who had designed the IMP 15 years before).

Any method of expired-air collection entails carrying a rubber or plastic mouthpiece, wearing a noseclip or plugs (or wearing a face mask or hood) and carrying Douglas bags or other measuring/sampling devices. No one is able or willing to undergo this for long periods, and the analysis of many gas samples, by whatever means, can be a tedious job. Despite this, these methods have been used for measuring the energy cost of many different sorts of occupation, from lying asleep to work at the coalface or strenuous athletic pursuits. If people can keep an accurate diary of their daily activities, it is possible, by referring to results of these studies, to determine approximately their daily energy expenditure.

A completely different indirect method of measuring metabolic rate has recently been adapted for human use. The oxygen and the hydrogen atoms of water can be labelled with stable, or nonradioactive, isotopes ^2H and ^{18}O. Ingested in a small drink of labelled water, these isotopes remain in harmless but measurable amounts in the body for several weeks. Some of the labelled oxygen becomes part of carbon dioxide and is excreted in the breath, or as bicarbonate in the urine, along with labelled water. By measuring both labels in the urine the observer can determine carbon dioxide production rates and thence heat production rates. The human subjects can thus continue their normal living habits, apart from the periodic collection of a urine sample, while their metabolic rates are being determined.

The energy output of the living body

Since virtually all of the energy lost from a living organism is heat energy (apart from small components in excreted nitrogenous waste products and in external mechanical work – both of which are easily measured in studies of this subject), it is usual to think of it in terms of heat energy and measure it as such. The phrase *direct calorimetry* means just that – direct measurement of heat.

Components of energy output

It is conventional to speak of two components. The first is the basal metabolic rate (BMR), the metabolic turnover needed to maintain the many organs and tissues of the body when they are completely at rest. The second is the energy output required for such activities as digestion and absorption of food, the muscular activity required in postural maintenance or for exercise, and the metabolic activity needed to regulate body temperature.

While the second component is bound to vary a great deal within one person from time to time as well as between different people, the BMR has traditionally been thought to be a constant value, dependent only upon such factors as age, sex, body surface area and active cell mass. However, when the metabolic rate under 'basal' or postabsorptive conditions is actually measured, it is found to be variable. It is true that for any one person there is an average value around which repeated observations are scattered, provided the person's life style, food intake and amount of exercise remain constant. There is also an average value for an homogenous group of people when their metabolic rates are measured under controlled standardized conditions, but again the MRs of the members of this group will be scattered around the average value.

The term 'basal metabolic rate' is therefore sometimes replaced by 'thermogenesis'; this means 'heat production', carrying also the implication of regulatable heat production. Even so, the concept of basal rate is still widely used and forms the basis of calculations of energy expenditure; it cannot yet be rejected.

One of the causes of variation in thermogenesis in a person at rest in a comfortable environment is the food intake. Digestion and absorption of any foodstuff leads to a raised metabolic rate and so to raised heat production. It was once thought that protein foods had a specific effect in this matter and the term 'specific dynamic action' was coined. More accurate measurements have shown that there is no such effect peculiar to protein foods, but that all food ingestion has what is now called its 'thermic effect'.

The second way in which food intake affects heat production is that changing the energy content of the food produces parallel (but usually smaller) changes in thermogenesis. The experimental basis for this comes from studies on rats encouraged to overeat by being offered a wide variety and unlimited amounts of foods attractive to rats. Their extra food intake was found to be matched by extra heat production, so that no surplus was left over that might have been deposited in the animals' adipose tissue stores.

The site of the extra heat production was found to be in the 'brown fat' adipose tissue of the animals. This is found in many species of mammal, chiefly in the newborn and young animals, but in some species it persists as a recognizable entity into adulthood.

Brown fat is characterized by a brownish appearance to the naked eye. On microscopic examination the adipocytes contain more cytoplasm, enzymes and mitochondria (the site of oxidative metabolism) than do those of normal fat tissue. In one key factor, metabolic activity in brown fat differs from that of all other living tissues. It is unable to trap any of the energy released in oxidation in the 'high energy' containing compounds, adenosine triphosphate or creatine phosphate. All of the energy is converted immediately into heat energy and none is made available for chemical reactions or for external mechanical work. Metabolic activity in this tissue is stimulated by the sympathetic nervous system, by its neurotransmitter, noradrenaline, and by adrenaline, secreted normally by the adrenal glands when stimulated by their sympathetic nerves. It is proposed that a raised food intake stimulates the sympathetic nerves and so causes the raised

Table 3.3 Daily basal energy output, related to both sex and weight for adults.

Weight (kg)	Energy turnover (MJ per day)	
	Men	Women
45		4.6
50	5.6	5.0
55	6.0	5.4
60	6.5	5.9
65	6.9	6.3
70	7.3	6.7
75	7.6	7.1
80	8.0	7.4

metabolic activity in the brown adipose tissue. Perhaps the 'satiety' centres in the hypothalamus of the brain are implicated in this stimulation of sympathetic nerves.

Despite all this elegant work on the laboratory rat, it is not yet justified to apply all these findings to humans. Some supporting evidence has been obtained for food-induced increases in heat production, but since no identifiable brown fat exists in adults, and sympathetic stimulation leads only to release of fat into the bloodstream, the question must remain open. The evidence, when we look at well-fed human populations such as that of the United Kingdom, is that thermogenesis only partly compensates for changes in food energy intake and at least some of the excess food gets deposited in the body's fat tissue stores.

The resting metabolic rate is frequently determined from a measurement of O_2 uptake using a recording spirometer, assuming an RQ of 0.85 and negligible protein metabolism, or an energy equivalent of 20 kJ per litre of O_2. Basal metabolism or thermogenesis at rest is now expressed as kJ heat produced per kg body weight; which for most people has been found to be a reasonable approximation to the active cell mass of the living body. This is the mass of actively metabolizing tissue; in other words, the whole body, less the deposits of fat, the crystalline material of bone and relatively noncellular connective tissues, tendons and ligaments. It is far harder to determine active cell mass than body weight.

Table 3.3 shows what the BMR ought to be, in MJ for people of different weights. The phrase 'ought to be' really should read: 'is found, on average, in healthy, well-fed but not overweight people to be'. A wide range of individual variation of 10% to 15% of this average value exists on both sides of the average. Basal metabolism also declines with age, and for any age is about 10% lower in females than in males.

Table 3.4 shows equations that have been derived for the determination of BMR from body weight for each of six age ranges. These ranges have been chosen to represent periods of life which differ in physiological or functional aspects. Equations for male and female BMRs are shown separately. In the elderly and children under 3 years old the inclusion of height would improve the prediction of BMR. Knowledge of the BMR is important medically in detection of certain disease states. In human nutrition its importance is that it gives us a jumping-off point below which a person's daily total metabolism can never fall and below which, therefore, the energy content of the food eaten cannot fall without eventual harm.

Table 3.4 Equations for predicting basal metabolic rate in MJ per day from body weight (*W*) in kg. From FAO/WHO/UNU (1985) *Energy and Protein Requirements*

Age (years)	Males	Females
0–3	$0.26W - 0.23$	$0.26W - 0.21$
3–10	$0.095W + 2.1$	$0.094W + 2.1$
10–18	$0.073W + 2.7$	$0.051W + 3.1$
18–30	$0.064W + 2.8$	$0.062W + 2.1$
30–60	$0.049W + 3.7$	$0.036W + 3.5$
Over 60	$0.057W + 2.0$	$0.044W + 2.5$

For the average adult European male this is about 7.0 MJ/day. He needs therefore at least 7.0 MJ in his food each day if he is merely to exist and not actually do anything, even eat, digest and absorb this food! If any man's average food intake contains less than 7.0 MJ/day, then he will probably be undernourished.

Daily energy needs

The energy output of nonbasal activities, whether these be engendered by work or by leisure-time pursuits, can be estimated from expired-air analysis techniques. Combined with a timetable of daily activities, these can be used to estimate the total daily energy outputs of people who are living their normal lives. The direct measurement of heat output from a person living in the human calorimeter gives a far more accurate figure for daily energy output, but the range of activities is greatly restricted.

It is largely the material gained from indirect studies of energy outputs ('basal' metabolism plus energy cost of activities) that provides us with a figure for the food energy requirements of people, since energy intake must, if the system is to remain stable, equal energy output.

The more advanced textbooks of nutrition contain tables derived from Food and Agriculture Organization/World Health Organization estimations of energy needs showing the estimated average energy needs of people in various occupations, and the energy needs of their leisure-time activities. One such estimate is given in Table 3.5. The figures shown are people's outputs. Allowing for a 5% loss from wastage at table, this means that their energy input (in their food) must be higher per day on average than these figures.

Similar calculations, based on respiratory gas analyses and accurate daily activity records, are used to determine the required intake for all sorts and conditions of men, women and children. Comparison of these – in individuals, groups or

Table 3.5 Typical estimate of an individual's energy output.

	Sedentary (MJ)	Moderate activity (MJ)	Heavy work (MJ)
Basal metabolism for 8 hours' rest in bed	2.0	2.0	2.0
Metabolism for leisure-time activities	3.0–7.0	3.0–7.0	3.0–7.0
Metabolism for 8 hours' work	4.0	5.5	7.5
Total	9.0–13.0	10.5–14.5	12.5–16.5

Table 3.6   The recommended daily energy intake for the UK.

	Age	MJ			MJ
Children	0–1	3.3	Men	Sedentary	11.1
	1–3	5.5		Moderately active	12.4
	3–7	7.1		Very active	15.1
	7–9	8.8		Retired	9.3
Boys	9–12	10.5	Women	Most occupations	9.2
	12–15	11.7		Very active	10.5
	15–18	12.6		55–75 years old	8.6
Girls	9–18	9.6		3–9 months pregnant	10.0
				Lactating	11.3

even whole nations – with the food available and consumed, determines their energy nutritional status.

Scales of energy needs

These are prepared by official bodies, taking (it is hoped) expert advice, and (it is equally hoped) used in policy decisions by government and other organizations. The one quoted here, in Table 3.6, is drawn from the British Department of Health and Social Security (DHSS), published by them in 1979. This table differs from the American NAS table shown in the first two editions of this book, the American table tending to be more generous, particularly in the first year of life and in the teens.

Such a table represents the *average* requirements for each group, and should never be applied in hard and fast ways to individual people. Nor should such a table be regarded as immutable truth, to apply for all time. It is the best estimate, made in the late seventies by a panel of experts with considerable practical experience in many fields, using the evidence then available. It can be used in the following ways.

If a group of people – say in an institution – is taking a diet within a range of plus or minus 10% of the appropriate estimated need, their diet may be considered satisfactory, so far as energy is concerned. This is where the 'housekeeping method' of dietary survey is used, and one must be aware of the errors liable to occur in this method. Thus in one such survey in a school, the energy intake during the test period was found to be well above the estimated requirement. It was assumed the school's catering manager, in order to impress his observers, had deliberately saved up foods from previous weeks in order to put on a good show during the test period!

In smaller groups – a family, for example – the individual diet survey method is used. An example is shown in Table 3.7, and the observed values can be compared with the DHSS estimates. Care must be taken in applying the DHSS recommendations, since people do differ so much both in their basal rates of thermogenesis and in their daily activities.

While it seems, from a first glance at the total figures, that all is well, when one looks at individual members of the family, some anxiety may be felt. Both parents are eating well above their estimated needs. Are they overweight, or more active

Table 3.7 Actual energy intakes for a family.

	DHSS estimate (MJ)	Actual consumption (MJ)
Father (bank manager)	11.1	13.0
Mother (moderately active)	9.2	10.8
Daughter 16 years old	9.6	5.0
Son 11 years old	10.5	9.0
Daughter 9 years old	8.8	9.2
Total	49.2	47.0
Total by Housekeeping Method		51.0

than their job descriptions state? For instance, the bank manager may be a keen landscape gardener in his spare time and his wife an energetic sportswoman. Then the actual intake of the 16-year-old daughter gives cause for concern. Is this an expression of the anxiety over examinations that upsets many of her age group? Is she having 'boyfriend trouble' or is she suffering from anorexia nervosa (a compulsive state in which the person – usually a 'high achiever', late-teenaged girl – refuses to eat an adequate amount of food)?

There is such a wide range of actual intake in normal healthy people, that it is only when the discrepancy between the observed intake and the estimated requirement exceeds 20% of the estimate (it was 30% in the 16-year-old girl just quoted) that further investigation is needed. Studies of large numbers of actual intakes, to obtain a reliable estimate of spontaneous variation, are very tedious to perform.

Such a study was made by Bingham and her colleagues in 1977. Sixty-three adults were randomly selected from the electoral register of a Cambridgeshire village. Their age and social class ranges were the same as those of the general population and the sample contained 32 males and 31 females. The foods they ate were weighed over a seven-day period and the energy contents calculated from the recorded weights. The average intake for the men was 10.0 MJ/day and for the women it was 8.2 MJ/day. These averages, however, are based on very wide ranges. The highest intake among the men was about 15.6 MJ and the lowest about 5.5 MJ. The corresponding figures for the women were 12.2 MJ and 3.0 MJ. Although the groups were small, both sets of results show no marked deviation from a normal distribution of individual results about the two average values. While about 40% of the whole group were conscious of the need to 'watch their weight', two of the overweight women consumed 9 and 11 MJ/day.

All these figures give lower values then those obtained in the 1930s by McCance and Widdowson and various studies in intervening years, which have all shown a gradual but persistent decline in this 50-year period. This may be attributed to an increased awareness of the problems of being overweight, or to decreasing demands on energy expenditure that follow the more widespread use of labour-saving devices, central heating, spectator rather than participatory leisure activities, etc. The conflicting effects of all these aspects of our life style have not, however, prevented 45% of the men and 40% of the women in Bingham's sample from being detectably overweight.

Obesity

Before we can discuss the relationship between food intake, body weight and fat stores, metabolic rate, and the significance of being overweight, it is necessary to have a meaningful scale of what we mean by 'overweight'. Many indices of this have been devised. The one that combines the greatest ease of measurement with the greatest nutritional and medical significance is the *body mass index*. This is a person's weight in kilograms divided by height in metres squared (W/H^2, in kg/m^2). Indices range (for adults) from below 20 to above 40. Mild obesity is defined as being present in a person with an index between 25 and 30, moderate obesity is between 30 and 40, and severe obesity is present when the index is above 40. The division between normality and mild obesity at an index of 25 is based partly on the Metropolitan Life Insurance tables of mortality and a critical re-appraisal of them by Dr Garrow in 1979. Distribution curves of W/H^2 for various groups in a north-west London suburb are shown in Fig. 3.4. It can be seen that

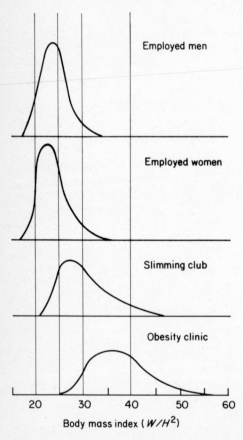

Fig. 3.4   Distribution of W/H^2 among employed men, employed women, members of a slimming club, and patients attending a hospital obesity clinic in Harrow, England. Redrawn from Garrow (1981).

for employed men the curve is symmetrical about its average (the peak of the curve), which is at an index of 24. Thus nearly half this sample are obese to some extent. Employed women have a peak lower than that for men, but their curve has a distinct tail at the obese end. The other two groups have higher average indices and even greater numbers in the higher levels of obesity.

What put these people where they are on these distribution curves, and what are their present food energy intakes and metabolic rates? One can only assume that the food energy intake has exceeded energy output and that, unlike the overeating rats, the excess energy has been stored in the body as fat. If, in the established state, one examines both metabolic rate and food intake, one finds that overweight people are in balance. Furthermore one finds that their basal metabolic rates, calculated on the standard of unit mass of active cells, are quite normal. Adipose tissue itself is living tissue; every 400 g of fat is contained in cells with about 100 g of actively metabolizing cytoplasm. In addition, the body systems that 'serve' this tissue – the heart and circulation, the lungs and other organs – all have to work harder or metabolize more than they would if the adipose tissue were not there. Thus the several kilograms of adipose tissue carried by an obese person contribute significantly to his or her metabolic heat production.

An equally important fact is that adipose tissue may accumulate slowly over several years. A daily imbalance between intake and needs of only 1%, if it were all to be deposited as fat, would result in the accumulation of 1.0 kg of adipose tissue in a year. At this rate of weight gain, the body mass index would increase in a decade by 3.5 units.

In biological systems with no emotional, social or cultural influences operating it is rare to find such a precise degree of homeostasis as is implied by the 1% imbalance figure used in this calculation. Larger discrepancies will develop, due to the individual and social/psychological factors which affect food intake and thus increase the imbalance. This leads both to the common state of a body mass index of above 25 and to the more rare state, anorexia nervosa, in which energy intake is less than the body's requirements and the weight falls, giving a body mass index markedly below 20. This imbalance is also distressingly common in those many parts of the world where food supply is insufficient to meet normal metabolic need.

As has been mentioned before, food has a thermic effect, and deprivation of food has the converse effect. Immediately following a reduction in energy intake, the daily heat output falls. This fall is variable in extent; in some people it may be almost as large as the fall in food energy intake and such people will lose weight very slowly. In others, more fortunately, metabolic rate falls only slightly in response to the reduction in food intake. They call upon their adipose tissue to a much greater extent in making up the deficit. Reduction of adipose tissue mass also causes a fall in metabolic rate, for the cytoplasmic fraction of adipose tissue atrophies as its fat is removed, and the 'service' demands made by the adipose tissue on other body systems fall. So the less one eats, the less one needs to eat. It is small wonder, then, that weight reduction by dietary restriction is so difficult to achieve.

The effects of obesity are clearly seen in Fig. 3.5, relating obesity to mortality. The actual links between increased body weight and death are varied and of varying degrees of directness. Obesity is directly linked with type II or maturity-onset diabetes mellitus. While a well-controlled diabetic person may not die from the

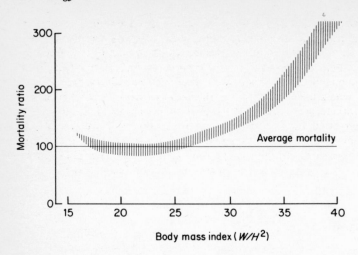

Fig. 3.5   Relation of body mass index (W/H^2) to mortality ratio. Redrawn from Garrow (1981).

disease or its complications, diabetic control is not always well maintained and diabetes is 5 to 8 times more common as a cause of death in the obese than in non-obese people. Being overweight means that more physical work or metabolic energy is needed for all daily activities, even lying in bed. This draws upon the cardiovascular and respiratory reserves all the time. Failure, usually of the heart, is the end result of such continuous overload. Obesity is also associated with a raised arterial blood pressure and with artery wall disease (atheroma), both of which reduce life expectancy. Finally, hip and knee joints are more likely to develop osteoarthritis due to the increased load on them. While this may not directly reduce lifespan, the resultant inactivity renders the body less resistant to other diseases, and it increases the risk of accidental falls.

Treatment of obesity

Treatment of obesity centres on two concepts. One is the prevention or early arrest of its development. A rise in the body mass index towards or past 25, growth of 'middle-age spread' or the 'beer pot' indicates that energy intake is in excess of energy needs. Some simple dietary restriction, such as eliminating beer, or sugar in hot drinks, coupled with increasing exercise, may arrest the spread before it gets too far.

The other concept, applied in treating established obesity, is simply that the energy content of the food eaten must be reduced to well below the daily energy needs of the body, and kept below the needs as these reduce. This must not, though, reduce the intake of essential food factors other than energy. Thus the protein, water-soluble and fat-soluble vitamins, minerals and fibre must be present in the required amounts, even though the energy content of the food is reduced.

First eliminate the 'empty energy' – foods that add energy alone. Sweet biscuits, cakes and pastry must go. Grilling should replace frying. Fatty meats should be replaced with lean cuts. Alcoholic drinks, especially those containing free sugar or dextrins, must be restricted. In all these ways, foods supplying excessive energy can be reduced, and it is quite simple to produce a diet containing only 4 MJ or 1000 kcals/day without affecting its protein, vitamin or other components. This may not be low enough in energy content for those with a good negative thermogenic effect – in whom metabolic turnover declines as energy intake is reduced. They, and many others, are tempted to try periods of more drastic food reduction, even complete starvation, for days or weeks at a time. This has its dangers. Stores of the water-soluble B vitamins are easily depleted, and even the store of ascorbic acid, potentially capable of supporting a person for three months, may be low at the start of a fast. Once any of these stores are emptied, problems ensue.

Undernutrition

Although the major nutritional problem in the United Kingdom is that of excessive consumption, in many other parts of the world people cannot get enough to eat. We in the UK are also seeing an increase in the frequency of anorexia nervosa, a self-starvation condition that shows, on the psychological side, some of the aspects of an obsessive-compulsive state.

In undernutrition or starvation, the important lack is of both protein and energy. For a poor person, an energy-low diet is bound to be low in protein content, since the cheaper and more easily produced foods are starch-containing foods with only 1 to 10% protein (and these proteins are deficient in one or more essential amino acids). To satisfy the protein need by, for example, supplementing food intake with a drink made from skimmed milk power without also meeting the energy needs is useless, since the protein will be used as an energy source. So long as food intake is energy or protein deficient, body proteins will be used both as an energy source and to provide essential amino acids. These points have already been made in the discussion on the planning of the diet for reducing obesity.

Deficiencies in food intake of the micronutrients (minerals and vitamins) will also inevitably occur when protein/energy malnutrition is present. Since micronutrient deficiencies can also occur in diets adequate in both major factors, they are described in the later chapters of this book.

If we compare the scales of energy and protein needs that are accepted throughout the world with the figures of actual food availability, we see that at least half of the world's population suffers from a marked energy deficit, and that less than a quarter obtain a food intake that is really adequate. Moreover, due to improved medical care, particularly since the 1940s, the rate of population increase may actually exceed the rate at which food production rises. Furthermore, the increases in food production that have been achieved have been obtained by using exhaustible reserves of mineral fertilizer and fossil fuels, and at the expense of soil quality and tree cover in many marginal and arid regions of the earth's surface. Optimists believe that we can overcome these problems, aided by a strict application of birth-control measures.

Whatever we may think of the future, the scales do provide clear evidence, here and now, of extremely widespread undernutrition in the world.

Anorexia nervosa

This condition seems to be increasing in frequency in the 1970s and 1980s, and has produced much discussion about its social, psychological and possible physical causes, as well as about its physical effects and treatment. It arises in people during adolescence, usually in girls who are expected to do well in academic school-leaving examinations by their parents. Frequently the victims become obsessed about their weight, physical appearance or the development of sexual maturity. Some have suggested that the condition is a symbolic retreat from adulthood to the infantile state, or that it is the result of the present fashions in physical build considered right for the young adult female.

The condition, leading to insufficient intake of foods, produces the same end-effects as does an inadequate food supply. All the foregoing discussion of protein/energy deficiency and of vitamin shortages applies equally well to anorexia. One feature that receives special attention in anorexia is the effect on the menstrual cycle. Ovulation and menstruation cease, and the regular cyclic changes in the hypothalamus and pituitary gland function are found to be absent. Recovery of this activity may be delayed for months or even years after the obsessive self-starvation regime has been broken and the sufferer has regained a normal body weight and protein content. This persistence of a physical aspect of the disease has led some to suggest that it is primarily a disturbance of the 'appetite centres' of the hypothalamus, which are close to those controlling the menstrual cycle. However, this view takes no account of the striking similarities in personal, familial and social backgrounds of those who develop anorexia. Such psychological and social considerations are beyond the scope of this book. However, they are well described in *The Art of Starvation* by Sheila McLeod, published in 1981 by Virago.

4
Carbohydrates

In this and in the next two chapters, we describe the chemistry, digestion and uses in the living body of carbohydrates, proteins and fats. However, certain general points must first be made about the digestive system.

Digestion

Most of the foods which we eat are insoluble in water. The body is at least 60% water, and the tissues where the chemical activities subserving life take place are at least 70% water, and it is in this water that those activities take place. Consequently food must be rendered water-soluble. Solubility, however, is not enough. Egg-white proteins are soluble in water, but they will not diffuse through animal cell membranes. Their molecules are too large. If made smaller they would become diffusible. But even diffusibility is not enough. Cane sugar is diffusible through cell membranes; nonetheless cane sugar, if it gets into the blood stream, is of no use to the body. It is excreted at once in the urine. Each substance in the food has to become usable by the body cells – call it 'metabolizable'.

To render foods soluble, diffusible and 'metabolizable' the body uses the alimentary tract, a set of tubular organs passing from mouth to anus, a part of the external world tucked into and through the body, some 6.5 m long in the dead body, but in life, such is its tone and elasticity, only 2.7 m long. The functions of this tract are partly mechanical and partly chemical – the food has to be broken up physically into smaller and smaller pieces, and also, chemically, into simpler and simpler compounds. To bring about the physical changes there is the grinding apparatus of the teeth; further along the tract contractions of its muscular wall aid breaking up food and mixing it with the chemical digestive agents. All these processes are together called digestion.

The term 'indigestion'

This has two very different meanings. The physiologist means by 'indigestible' a foodstuff which the enzymes in the gut cannot change to simpler substances, and which cannot therefore be absorbed. Some indigestible food materials may be attacked by the bacteria normally resident in the lower parts of the gut, which then produce gases; carbon dioxide, methane or hydrogen. These, if not absorbed into the blood, distend the gut.

'Indigestion' to the physician means pain arising from the gut consequent upon taking food. Gaseous distension is one cause of pain. Over-activity in the gut's muscle wall is another. Oversecretion of acid by the stomach is a third. In the latter two cases, the fault lies not with the digestibility of the food eaten, but in the reactions of the gut to foods.

Digestive enzymes

To produce complete chemical digestion of foodstuffs the alimentary tract produces a whole battery of enzymes, each one catalysing a single chemical reaction. Generic names for enzymes end in '-ase': protease for protein-splitting, lipase for fat-splitting, sucrase for cane sugar-splitting enzymes, and so on. Often enzymes will be given specific names – as it were first names – e.g. the protease of the gastric secretion is called pepsin.

These enzymes may be secreted into the lumen of the gut and mixed with the food, or they may be retained within the surface membrane of its lining and complete digestion after partly broken down and soluble food products have been absorbed.

The secretion of enzymes into the gut is a controlled process, only occurring when food is eaten. The control mechanisms are partly nervous and partly chemical. Some are true reflexes, stimulated by the sight, smell or taste of the food (an obvious example is the secretion of saliva). Food products in the gut may cause the release, from its lining cells into the blood, of substances that stimulate the glands that produce the digestive enzymes. These substances belong to the class of regulatory chemicals called hormones, or chemical messengers.

Mouth

The chief function of the mouth is the breaking up of the food into small pieces convenient to swallow. This is done by the combined action of teeth and tongue. Thorough chewing of food is important, since this mixes it, in small particles, with the watery saliva which enables subsequent mixing of food and digestive enzymes to occur more easily in the stomach and intestine. Saliva contains mucus which coats the food with a slippery layer and makes it easier to swallow.

The volume of saliva varies with the condition of the body, and the nature and taste of the food. A thirsty person cannot produce saliva readily, which should be remembered when feeding a dehydrated person. Wet food evokes less saliva than dry food, but the most potent factor in producing saliva is the taste or smell of food. Acidity always evokes salivation, as does astringency. If the food is liked or the person is hungry the flow of saliva is greatest. Saliva keeps the mouth clean. Any feverish illness reduces saliva production, so not only is swallowing difficult, but the mouth may become dirty and even infected.

The food, when sufficiently chewed and mixed with saliva, is swallowed and passes down the oesophagus (which has no other function than being a connecting tube) to the stomach. Here it is retained for 1 to 5 hours, or even longer.

Stomach

The practical convenience of having a reservoir early in the alimentary tract is obvious. Its capacity determines how often a person has to eat. It varies much between individuals, but is generally not enough for the one-meal-a-day person, and 'little and often' is the best rule in taking meals.

The stomach's secretion depends on both nervous and chemical controls. Sensory receptors in the nose and tongue reflexly stimulate the stomach as soon as food is eaten, and this persists as long as the meal is enjoyed. The more the food (and its setting) is liked, the greater the flow of secretion and, presumably, the better the digestion. Some foods (e.g. meat extracts and meat-derived soups) set free from the stomach lining the hormone *gastrin*, which further stimulates the secretory activity. Other foods when partly digested have the same effect. Reflexly produced secretion contains both acid and enzymes, but gastrin-evoked secretion contains mostly acid. The acid is hydrochloric acid and its maximal strength is about 0.1 M or about 0.35%. The total amount secreted will depend upon the interaction of other nervous activity with the reflexes described, upon the nature of the foods eaten, and upon other factors in the individual person. Some people secrete more acid and others little or even no acid. If either extreme is producing trouble appropriate feeding should be instituted, based on foods which such a person can tolerate.

The concentration of hydrochloric acid in the stomach is normally sufficient to kill any disease-causing bacteria present in the food. This accounts for the fact that not everyone who ingests food or water contaminated with food-poisoning bacteria is poisoned, and why it is particularly dangerous to drink infected water on an empty stomach.

Mixing of food and secretion is produced by contractions of the stomach's muscular wall. The organ is U-shaped, with the right limb of the U shorter than the left. The left limb remains largely quiescent, its walls behaving as an elastic bag would do on filling. In the right limb rings of contraction appear, moving slowly up towards the pylorus at its distal end. These rings of contraction gently massage and mix the various contents of the stomach. The sphincter at the pylorus is normally contracted and closes the stomach, preventing its contents from entering the small intestine. However, the contraction rings moving over the stomach's wall raise its internal pressure and eventually force its macerated and liquid contents through the sphincter.

Small intestine

The secretions of the small intestine and of the liver and pancreas, and the digestive enzymes found in the lining cells of the intestinal wall, are described later. Here it should be noted that components of the food that leave the stomach cause the liberation from the duodenal wall of two further hormones, secretin and pancreozymin, which stimulate secretion of the pancreas and contraction of the gall bladder. The total 24-hour volume of all secretions poured into the gut approaches 10 litres. All this has to be reabsorbed as the mixture passes further along the small intestine.

The most important muscular activity of the small intestine is that of segmental contraction and relaxation. Short segments of the gut's muscle contract, while intervening segments relax, respectively emptying and filling the contracted and relaxed segments. Then the relaxed segments contract, and vice versa. This process continually mixes the contents of the intestine, exposing food products to digestive enzymes and the absorbing surface of the gut.

Bulk movement of contents from the stomach towards the terminal ileum and thence into the colon may also be assisted by these sequential contractions if they occur with a short time delay from above (stomach end) downwards (towards ileal termination). It is, however, just as likely that entry of food from the stomach, and digestive secretions from liver and pancreas, together with absorption further down the small intestine, causing distension above and collapse below, provide the mechanical forces needed to drive the contents along the small intestine.

Large intestine

Secretion by the wall of the large intestine or colon is confined to mucus, which protects its lining cells and lubricates the contents which eventually become semi-solid due to water absorption. In the colon, while segmental mixing continues, large-scale bulk movement of contents by peristalsis is also seen. Peristalsis is a contraction that begins at one of the colon and sweeps progressively along the muscle, driving the colonic contents before it. Such contractions may be reflexly stimulated by the presence of food in the stomach, as well as by the quantity of material entering the colon from the small intestine, or by gas formed in the colon by its resident bacteria. These micro-organisms live on the indigestible and unab-sorbed residues of the food, converting this material progressively into their own cell bodies. These residues are loosely called 'dietary fibre', consisting largely of various polysaccharide materials (see page 50). Their bulk, and that of the bacterial bodies they sustain, is a direct result of their content in the food eaten. In this way the quantity of fibre eaten directly affects the motility of the colon and rate of passage of food through it. People whose diet has a high fibre content suffer less from various diseases of the colon than others, although the cause-effect links are not yet known. High-fibre diets also may slow the rate of glucose and fat absorp-tion from the small gut and thus reduce the liability to develop diabetes and arterial disease (rapid rises of blood glucose and fat in the absorption period after meals respectively being among their causative factors).

The long-standing belief that the large intestinal contents should be kept regu-larly on the move may therefore be partly true. However, the advice of the patent medicine advertisers on the use of medicinal purgative or laxative substances is almost certainly false. What is needed is to raise the fibre content of the diet from around 20 grams to over 30 grams per day. This will bring about the beneficial results thought to be associated with a high-fibre diet.

Conclusion

This brief survey of secretory and motor functions of the gut has deliberately not included any description of the digestive and absorptive processes affecting the nutritional components of our food. These are described sequentially, in this chapter for carbohydrates and in the next four chapters for fats, proteins, minerals and vitamins respectively.

The chemistry of carbohydrates

Carbohydrates are a group of compounds of the elements carbon, hydrogen, and oxygen. The latter two are present in the same proportion (two atoms of hydrogen to one of oxygen) as in water; hence the name carbohydrate, for *hudor* is the Greek for water. Carbohydrates are found in food either as sugars or as polysaccharides. These latter materials are long, straight or branched chains of many sugar molecules joined together. The chemical nature of the sugars determines their properties, their function in living tissues and how they are formed and broken down.

Monosaccharides

These are the simplest sugars known to the chemist and physiologist. Each molecule of these may consist of 4 or 5, but usually 6, carbon atoms, the same number of oxygen atoms and twice the number of hydrogen atoms. Usually sugar molecules exist in a ring form, the ring containing all but one of the carbon atoms and an oxygen atom. The remaining carbons, the hydrogen and the other oxygen atoms are placed 'above' or 'below' the ring. Glucose is a monosaccharide containing in each molecule 6 carbon, 12 hydrogen and 6 oxygen atoms. Thus it has an empirical formula $C_6H_{12}O_6$. An attempt to draw its three-dimensional molecular structure is shown in Fig. 4.1

Fructose and galactose are the other monosaccharides of major nutritional importance. They have the same empirical formula as glucose, but differ (as seen in Fig. 4.1) in the disposition of the accessory atoms and groups around the basic carbon and oxygen ring structure. These structural differences are of great importance once the monosaccharides enter the living body, for they determine the ways in which they can be used. These three ways of arranging the same carbon, hydrogen and oxygen atoms around the basic ring structure are not the only possible arrangements. Many other configurations are possible, and some exist in various plant and bacterial carbohydrates.

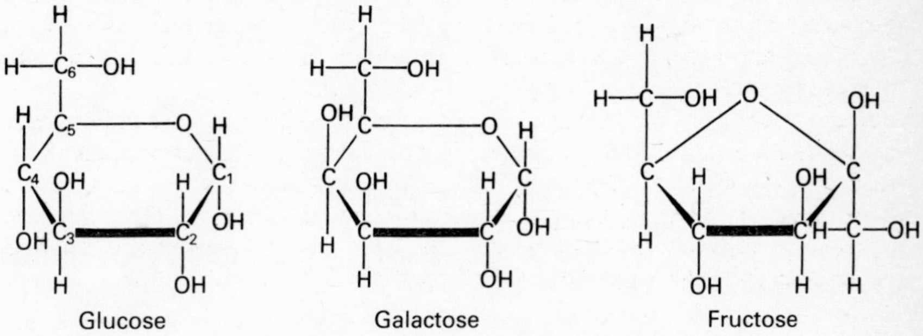

Fig. 4.1 Structural formulae for glucose, galactose and fructose.

Disaccharides

Monosaccharides readily combine into pairs known as disaccharides. Those of importance in nutrition are sucrose, formed from one molecule of glucose and one of fructose; lactose, formed from glucose and galactose; and maltose, formed from two glucose molecules. In each case a molecule of water is lost when the two monosaccharides combine, so the empirical formulae of disaccharide molecules is $C_{12}H_{22}O_{11}$.

Sugars and polarized light

Light beams behave as though the rays are vibrating transversely to the direction of the beam. Special optical apparatus can produce rays all vibrating in the same plane, known as polarized light. Solutions of compounds with asymmetry in their structure rotate the plane of vibration of light passing through them. All these monosaccharides are asymmetrical at carbons 1 to 4. Glucose rotates the plane of polarization in one direction, fructose more strongly in the opposite direction. When the two monosaccharides combine to form sucrose, this compound rotates light in the same direction as glucose.

Breaking sucrose down to a mixture of glucose and fructose thus results in an inversion of the rotation direction. Enzymes that cause this effect are known as invertases, and the resultant mixture of glucose and fructose is sometimes called 'invert sugar'.

Polysaccharides

These are chain molecules formed from many monosaccharides linked together. The chains can be straight or branched and can be formed from any of the 6-carbon monosaccharides already described, from 5-carbon sugars, or from the amino sugars, related compounds having an $-NH_2$ group in place of one of the $-OH$ groups. The only polysaccharides of major nutritional importance, because they can be digested in the human gut, are starches and glycogen (other polysaccharides are important as components of dietary fibre, see below).

Starches and glycogen are formed from chains of glucose molecules. Amylose is a straight-chain form of starch, containing several hundred glucose molecules, linked 'head to tail' between carbon 1 of one glucose molecule and carbon 4 of the next (as in maltose, a molecule of water is lost in forming the link). Amylopectin and glycogen are branched chains. In these a second link is formed, between carbon 6 of one unit and carbon 1 of another. These branches occur at 18 to 20 glucose unit intervals in glycogen, but at longer intervals in amylopectin. Many thousand glucose units may be present in a single branched-chain polysaccharide. In starch and glycogen the carbon 1–4 linked glucose units are all arranged the same way round, the links being known as alpha-1,4-glucosidic links.

In cellulose the 1,4 link is of the beta (β) type, in which adjacent glucose units are orientated at 180° to each other, so that alternate units are 'upside down'. Cellulose, like amylose, exists only as straight-chain molecules. This type of link cannot be hydrolyzed by any of our digestive system's amylases (more precisely called α-1,4-glucosidases).

Cellulose is the main structural component of all plant cell walls; associated with it are a heterogeneous collection of other branched-chain polysaccharides, formed from pentoses (monosaccharides with only 5 carbon atoms), galactose, amino sugars or acidic derivatives of glucose and galactose, collectively at one time called 'hemicelluloses'. Like cellulose, none of these can be digested by human digestive enzymes. Inulin is a storage form of polysaccharide formed from fructose by artichokes and related plants; agar from galactose, and various gums and mucilages including pectin come from different plant species. Collectively all these compounds are known as 'dietary fibre', though some are water-soluble and never fibrous. Lignin, though not a polysaccharide at all, is included as a component of dietary fibre because it comes from plant cell walls and is not digestible.

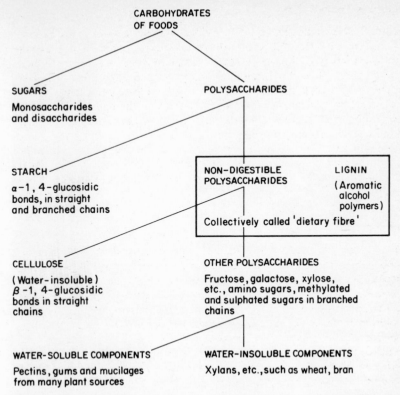

Fig. 4.2 Dietary fibre components and their relationship to digestible and absorbable carbohydrates.

The 'Maillard polymer', a compound formed when carbohydrates and proteins are cooked together in the browning process (i.e. in toast and other cooked cereal products), is also included in dietary fibre, since it is probably not broken down by digestive enzymes.

Dietary fibre reduces the rate of absorption of foodstuffs in the small gut and provides the food source for bacteria in the colon. In this process part of the material of fibre becomes the material of the bacteria. Short-chain fatty acids (Chapter 5) are also formed and may be absorbed. One of these, butyric acid, is an essential nutrient for the colon's lining cells. Both the fibre and the bacterial material increase the bulk of the gut contents (faeces) by their ability to absorb water and so prevent the colonic lining membrane from removing water from the faeces. This increase in bulk has the further effect of reducing the total time taken for material to pass through the gut. Figure 4.2 illustrates the classification of the different components of dietary fibre.

Occurrence of carbohydrates

Glucose appears to be the keystone of metabolism in both plants and animals. It is the main product of photosynthesis in green plants; however it is only rarely found free in plant material (grapes being the most significant exception). It is present in human blood, at about 80 to 120 mg/dl blood (5 to 6 mmol/litre), and is the only sugar that plays a major role in human metabolism. Fructose is found free in some fruits. Galactose occurs only in combination, as lactose, in milk.

Of the disaccharides, sucrose is widely distributed in plant fruits and in some other tissues (sugar cane and beet, and in maple syrup). It is, in fact, the common 'sugar' of regular daily use, our food sources being sugar cane and beet. Maltose is formed from the starch of grain seeds when they germinate. Lactose is secreted in mammalian milk.

Starch is the major storage form of carbohydrate found in plants, in seeds, root or stem stores, grain or pulses, root vegetables and potatoes. Glycogen is present in much smaller amounts (1 to 5%) in living muscle (meat) and liver etc., though much of this may be depleted in slaughtering and processing before consumption.

The sweetness of sugars lies principally in fructose. This is twice as sweet, molecule for molecule, as is sucrose, three times sweeter than glucose and eight times as sweet as lactose. Infants, perhaps, do not acquire a 'sweet tooth' as much from mother's milk as from sucrose added to or part of various proprietary infant foods.

Digestion and absorption of carbohydrates

Although the huge starch molecules can be very complicated, their building blocks are glucose molecules and only two types of link exist between the blocks. Therefore only a single type of enzyme, α-1, 4-glucosidase (amylase), is needed to effect almost their entire digestion. However, in raw foods starch comes in microscopic grains, each enclosed in a cellulose envelope. Only when cooking has destroyed this envelope can the digestive enzyme act on the starch and reduce it to the disaccharide maltose.

Salivary amylase will, while food is stored in the left-hand loop of the stomach, digest any cooked starch to dextrins (smaller polysaccharide molecules) and to maltose so long as the contents of that part of the stomach do not become markedly acid. Though this enzyme is accidental (most animals have it, though in a state of nature they do not eat cooked starch) it is as well to take advantage of it by eating starchy foods (puddings) late in the meal. Porous foods, such as rusks, are easily penetrable by saliva (whereas new bread is not), and therefore are easily digestible by salivary amylase.

The pancreatic amylase attacks unchanged cooked starch and dextrins and changes them to maltose. It is also said to digest uncooked starch, but with difficulty. Maltase carries on the digestion of maltose to glucose. Sucrase converts cane sugar into glucose and fructose. Lactase changes lactose to glucose and galactose. Lactase is present in the gut for the first two to three years in all human beings, but its production persists in adults of Caucasian races only. These people alone can therefore fully digest natural cows' milk, though all human beings can manage yoghurt or cheese in which the lactose has already been broken down by bacterial action. These three disaccharidases are found principally within the cells lining the gut.

When the digestible carbohydrates of the food have been converted by these enzymes to monosaccharides, the form in which they are metabolized, their absorption is actively completed by the small gut's lining cells. They diffuse down their concentration gradients through these cells, the spaces below them and so into the blood vessels of the gut wall. Both sodium ions (see Chapter 7) and water are absorbed along with the monosaccharides and about 95% of the available dietary carbohydrate is absorbed. Some of the glucose that escapes may be absorbed by the colon.

Carbohydrate metabolism

In discussing what happens to carbohydrates when they are metabolized in the body, it is simplest to consider glucose, fructose and galactose. They pass into the bloodstream, emerging from the intestines and perforce pass straight to the liver. All three are stored there as glycogen, but some of the glucose passes on (perhaps all of it) and is transformed into glycogen in the muscles. Ultimately the glycogen is shared between liver and muscles. Storage of glycogen is encouraged by insulin, the internal secretion of the pancreas. Liver glycogen is readily transformed back into glucose whenever the blood sugar level falls below 60–80 mg/dl (4 mmol/l), depending on the individual concerned. Fasting, cold and exercise deprive the liver of glycogen, but not the muscles. It passes into the bloodstream as glucose and is conveyed to the tissues – nervous system, glands and muscles – where it is consumed (oxidized) and energy obtained from this combustion. The final products of the combustion are carbon dioxide and water, but there may be more than one pathway (glycolysis and the 'pentose shunt' systems) used in the body. It is certain that the vitamins thiamine, riboflavin and nicotinic acid are concerned in cellular combustion of carbohydrate to carbon dioxide and water, and also that insulin is essential somewhere in the process. Carbohydrates can be converted into fat and stored; the proportion so treated depends on the person – and on the quantity eaten.

5
Fats

The fats are compounds of glycerol with fatty acids. Glycerol (also known commercially as glycerine), which is not unlike a 3-carbon sugar in structure, is commonly depicted as follows:

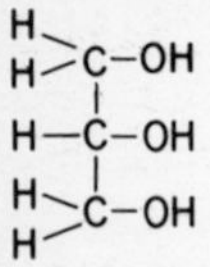

$$
\begin{matrix}
H \\
^{>}C-OH \\
H \\
| \\
H-C-OH \\
| \\
H \\
^{>}C-OH \\
H
\end{matrix}
\quad \text{or} \quad CH_2OH \,.\, CHOH \,.\, CH_2OH
$$

The fatty acids consist of chains of carbon and hydrogen atoms terminating at one end in the following acidic group

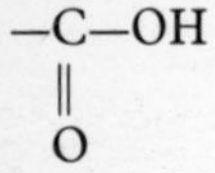

$$
\begin{matrix}
-C-OH \\
\| \\
O
\end{matrix}
$$

Butyric acid is thus

$$
\begin{matrix}
H & H & H \\
| & | & | \\
H-C-C-C-C-OH \\
| & | & | & \| \\
H & H & H & O
\end{matrix}
$$

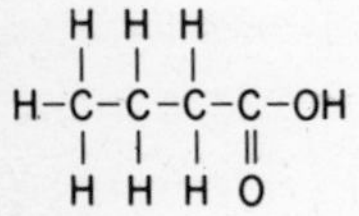

This formula is often abbreviated to $C_3H_7.COOH$. Sometimes there are double bonds between adjacent carbon atoms, with the loss of two hydrogen atoms:

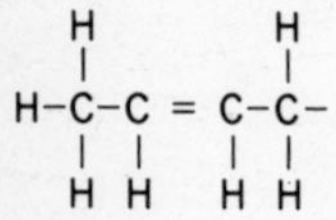

$$
\begin{matrix}
H & & H \\
| & & | \\
H-C-C & = & C-C- \\
| & | & | & | \\
H & H & H & H
\end{matrix}
$$

When a fatty acid combines with glycerol a water molecule is lost, thus:

$CH_2OH \,.\, CHOH \,.\, CH_2O \; \overline{[H + HO]} \; OC.C_3H_7 \rightarrow$

$CH_2OH \,.\, CHOH \,.\, CH_2O.OC.C_3H_7$ (glyceryl monobutyrate) $+ H_2O$

The dotted line indicating the water molecule lost.

Rarely in a complete fat is only one fatty acid present. Usually three different fatty acids are found attached to the glycerol molecule: in butter the main fat is glyceryl butyro-oleostearate, one molecule of each of the three acids being combined with the glycerol molecule. The final nature of a fat or oil, whether it be hard like lamb dripping, soft like butter, or liquid like vegetable oil, is determined by the fatty acids that are present in the fat.

Spontaneous chemical changes can take place in a fat. In the presence of water and some micro-organisms, the links between glycerol and the fatty acids can be split. The free acids may give an unpleasant taste, as when butter becomes rancid. Another change results from oxidation reactions at the site of the double bonds in the unsaturated fatty acids. Such reactions may, if uncontrolled, produce peroxide groupings which can have far-reaching and harmful effects upon living tissues.

Occurrence of fats

All living cells contain traces of fat in their structure, for fatty acids are among the components of cell wall and other intracellular membrane structures. In mammals and birds, fat deposits and stores are found throughout the body: between muscles, around internal organs and under the skin. Many fish have fat stored exclusively in the liver, but in the herring, for example, it is present throughout the flesh. In the vegetable kingdom, fats are found in the fruiting bodies of various plants, such as olives, maize, palm nuts, to name but a few.

Types of fatty acids

The carbon chain length of fatty acids can be from 2 to 22 or longer, though most have between 16 and 20 carbon atoms. Thus stearic acid contains 18 carbons, and palmitic acid has 16 carbons. Stearic acid is often written as $C_{17}H_{35}.COOH$ and palmitic acid as $C_{15}H_{31}.COOH$. Short-chain fatty acids – acetic, proprionic and butyric acids – are formed from bacterial decomposition of dietary fibre (the latter being found also in milk fat). In the longer fatty acids double valency bonds may be present between adjacent carbon atoms, these being known as unsaturated fatty acids. In oleic (18 C atoms) and palmitoleic (16 C atoms) acids only one such bond is present in the compound. They are therefore called monounsaturated fatty acids (MUFA). In others, such as linoleic acid (18 C atoms), more double bonds exist; these are polyunsaturated fatty acids (PUFA). These have a special significance in food in that they are essential in cell membranes and are the precursors of the prostaglandin compounds, important in many regulatory functions in the body; their presence in the food may protect partially against the development of arterial disease. None can be synthesized in the body, but all can be made from linoleic acid if this is in the food. This compound has two double bonds in the 18 carbon atom chain.

Two possible types of linkage of carbon to hydrogen atoms exist at a double bond. In the *cis* link, the hydrogen atoms are on the same side of the chain of carbon atoms, and cause the chain to be bent back on itself. In the *trans* form they are on opposite sides and the chain lies straight as do those of saturated fatty acids. It is only the former type of double bond that confers the essential quality to unsaturated fatty acids (Fig 5.1).

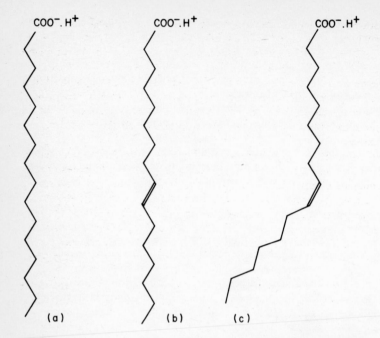

Fig. 5.1   Outline of the carbon atom chain's preferred states for **(a)** a saturated fatty acid, **(b)** *trans* form of mono-unsaturated fatty acid, and **(c)** *cis* form of mono-unsaturated fatty acid. Adding further double bonds of the *cis* type would cause the chain to double back. The *trans* type has no such effect.

Steroids

Associated with fats in foods are a group of compounds called steroids, which have a ring structure based on carbon and hydrogen atoms. The most important of these is cholesterol, an essential component of the fatty cell membranes, and also the precursor of many other substances essential to the body (including cholecalciferol or vitamin D – see Chapter 8). It is not surprising to find that we do not depend on foods for so important a substance. All the cholesterol the human body needs can be made in the liver. The significance of food cholesterol is that too much of the substance, that made by the liver plus that in the food, may be one of the several factors that together cause arterial wall disease, and thus strokes, heart attacks and gangrene.

Digestion and absorption of fats

As with polysaccharides, the chemistry of fats is relatively simple. One sort of lipase (fat-splitting enzyme) can split any link between glycerol and any fatty acid. There may be a lipase in the gastric secretion in infants, but the main lipase is that of the pancreas, which splits fats into fatty acids and glycerol in the jejunum. There is one problem, however, in this process. Fats are not soluble in the watery mixture of the small intestine, and would normally form large separate drops.

They can, however, be emulsified or split up into very small droplets by agents which are both fat-soluble and water-soluble. In the gut, it is the bile acids, compounds belonging to the steroid group, that emulsify the fat and so enable lipase to act. Bile acids are made in the liver from cholesterol, concentrated and stored in the bile ducts and gallbladder, and then added to the contents of the duodenum when food enters it from the stomach. Gallstones can block the secretion of bile into the gut; fat digestion is then greatly impaired and much of the fat in the food, together with fat-soluble vitamins, remains unabsorbed and is lost from the body in the faeces.

Partly split fats and free fatty acids aid the bile acids in emulsifying the neutral fats. It is not known how much of the neutral fat is broken down to free fatty acids or the intermediate compounds (monoglycerides and diglycerides). Particles of unsplit fat, partially hydrolyzed fat and free fatty acid can all be freely absorbed if the particle size is less than 0.5 micron. After absorption, 50 to 60% of the fat is found as unsplit fat in the lymphatics. Much of this may have been reconstituted by the cells in the intestinal wall. This fat consists of the long-chain fatty acids. The remainder (principally short-chain fatty acids) passes to the liver in the portal blood.

Bile acids themselves are reabsorbed in the ileum and pass in the blood to the liver, where they act as a stimulus for their resecretion into the bile. They thus undergo an *enterohepatic circulation*.

Metabolism of fat

The reconstituted fat molecules would, on their own, be insoluble in cell, interstitial, and plasma water. In the epithelium of the gut they are combined with special proteins to form *chylomicrons*. These are the largest and lightest of a group of compounds collectively known as lipoproteins. Lipoproteins are classified according to their density. At one end of the range are the large, light chylomicrons, then come very low density, low density and finally high density lipoproteins (VLDL, LDL and HDL).

As chylomicrons circulate in the blood, fats are removed from them by specific lipoprotein lipases in the blood vessel walls, especially in the liver, skeletal muscle and adipose tissue. From the fat it removes, the liver forms the VLDL and HDL fractions. LDL molecules are the residues left when chylomicrons have lost most of their fat in peripheral tissues. They contain the original cholesterol from the food and have further cholesterol freed by metabolism in all cells added to them.

Virtually all of the blood plasma cholesterol is present in LDL molecules. They are removed from the blood by specific receptor molecules in all tissues, but can also seep through the endothelial lining of arteries and be broken down by scavenger cells in the blood vessel wall. It is the products of this breakdown process that are thought to cause the common disease of arteries, atheroma. Excess food intake of fats containing cholesterol or saturated fatty acids, excess hepatic production of cholesterol, or scarcity of LDL receptor molecules are thus all possible causes of atheroma.

It is becoming clear that atheroma, a major factor in causing coronary arterial disease, strokes and gangrene in the legs, is itself a result of complex interaction between dietary fat and cholesterol intake, hepatic cholesterol synthesis, cholesterol metabolism in all other tissues of the body, and production of both LDL molecules and their specific receptors. Controlling dietary intake of fat and cholesterol is only one factor involved in atheroma prevention, but it is one that can be manipulated, for good or for ill, by determining what sort of food we eat. More saturated fatty acid in the diet causes increased production of LDL, but mono-unsaturated fatty acids raise the number of LDL receptors, while polyunsaturated fatty acids in the diet lower LDL concentration in the blood.

Adipose tissue

Any dietary fat not immediately taken into other tissues for oxidation (see below) is stored in adipose tissue, which it reaches in the original chylomicrons or as VLDL. This tissue can also take glucose from the blood and convert it into fat. The hormone insulin, liberated from the pancreas when glucose is being absorbed from the gut, stimulates both fat and glucose uptake by adipose tissue. Adipose tissue cells contain lipase molecules that are activated by hormones, particularly adrenaline and adrenal cortex hormones which are secreted in times of stress or exercise. The lipase splits the neutral fat and the fatty acids enter the blood plasma, become attached to albumin molecules and are transported thereon to other tissues for oxidative energy production. Muscles, whether at rest or exercising, use the oxidation of fat as their primary source of energy. It is only in more vigorous activity that carbohydrates provide their principal energy source.

Oxidation of fatty acids

Some of the fat that enters liver cells, whether from food or from adipose tissue, is oxidized by them, but some emerges as the partly oxidized fragments, beta-OH-butyric acid and acetoacetic acid, collectively known as ketone bodies.

Oxidation of fatty acids begins with successive splitting of acetic acid molecules from the end of the long-chain fatty acid molecules. These acetic acid molecules, in an active form, then enter the same common pathway that serves for carbohydrate oxidation. It is only when this pathway is depressed or blocked that active acetic acid molecules combine in pairs to form the ketone bodies. Fat oxidation becomes blocked and ketone bodies are produced if liver, muscle or other tissues do not have glycogen or glucose available for oxidation. A mild rise in ketone body production (ketosis) will occur whenever fat mobilization occurs, in exercise or in overnight fast or some condition associated with low food intake, such as an acute gastroenteritis or the nausea and vomiting of early pregnancy. A more severe ketosis, causing mental confusion or coma as well as physiological changes (muscular weakness and overbreathing) may occur in severe states of these kinds and also in diabetes mellitus, when insulin lack prevents normal glucose entry into cells and thus glucose oxidation. The symptoms usually thought to be associated with a mild ketosis – lethargy, headache and loss of appetite – are so common that it is unlikely that the association really exists, or that the ketosis is the cause of the symptoms.

Dietary requirement for fat

A fat-free diet is a dull one! Frying or roasting of foods produces flavours that cannot be obtained by boiling the same food. The higher temperatures produce the caramels and Maillard reaction products that we enjoy as flavours. Also, fats are a rich energy source and are easily eaten. It is not surprising, then, that diets in wealthy countries contain large amounts of fat. This, however, makes it easy to eat more than we need, so that the surplus is added to adipose tissue stores, and more LDL is formed, raising the incidence of arterial disease. Apart from the polyunsaturated fatty acids, we can synthesize in our own livers and adipose tissue all the varieties of fats and all the cholesterol we need from nonfatty precursors. The minimal amount of linoleic acid needed as the source of polyunsaturated fatty acids has not been established, but it might be as low as one gram per day.

Dietary fat is not even a particularly good source of the fat-soluble vitamins – common adipose tissue of beef, pork or lamb does not contain any of these – and the retinol or cholecalciferol present in dairy produce fats are only a minor source of these vitamins (see Chapter 8 for more on the fat-soluble vitamins).

Polyunsaturated fatty acids and cholesterol

In the 1960s many people began to accept the growing body of evidence that the unsaturated fatty acids were protective and that a high dietary intake of cholesterol was harmful. I am still not entirely convinced by the evidence for either statement. The level of cholesterol in the blood, which may have something to do with arterial disease, is only partly determined by the cholesterol in food, because no matter what our dietary intake, we make cholesterol in our own bodies. Foods high in cholesterol are eggs and brains. A high intake of saturated fatty acids raises plasma cholesterol, while increasing the intake of polyunsaturated fatty acids lowers plasma cholesterol. Most land animal fats, milk and its products ('every cow should carry a government health warning', some say!) and some vegetable oils contains mainly saturated fatty acids, whereas fish and other vegetable oils contain larger amounts of unsaturated fatty acids, as shown in Table 5.1.

Leaving aside the fatty fish (herrings, mackerel, salmon), we do not directly eat much of these polyunsaturated fats. They can be used as cooking fats, though on exposure to heat and air the double bonds are said by some to be readily oxidized.

Table 5.1 The fatty acid composition of some food fats (as a percentage of total fatty acids).

Food	C4–12 Saturated	C14–18 Saturated	C16+18 1 double bond	C18 2 double bonds	Others 2 or more double bonds	1 double bond
Milk etc.	11	47	36	4	1	
Beef		53	44	2		
Pork		34	44	21		
Fish oil		23	27	7	43	
Coconut oil	58	31	8	2		
Corn (maize) oil		15	31	53	1	
Ground nut oil		15	55	30		
Olive oil		16	71	10		
Palm oil		45	45	9		
Rape seed oil		4	16	14	9	50
Soya bean oil		14	24	53	7	
Sunflower seed oil		11	25	63		

They can be incorporated into margarine, and such margarine is now marketed. Attempts are also being made to enable those animals we rear for their meat to incorporate more polyunsaturated fatty acids in their depot fat. This can be done by feeding them vegetable material or fish meal containing the unsaturated fats; but in the interest of the global nutrition state, it would perhaps be better for these to be fed directly to humans.

To summarize, if it is accepted that a high blood cholesterol is harmful, then this can be increased by saturated fatty acids and reduced by polyunsaturated fatty acids. The former are present in meat, milk, palm and olive oils, the latter in fatty fish and the other vegetable oils in regular use. Their correct use in cooking and as a butter substitute is required if their intake is to be increased. Herring and mackerel, furthermore, must be protected from overfishing if their continued supply is to be maintained.

6
Proteins

The word *protein* is derived from Greek, and means 'holding the first place'. Proteins hold the first place in the architecture and machinery of all living things. Without them no life can exist. No plant can grow or trap sunlight, no baby can be born or reared, unless proteins have been made. There is an enormous range of proteins: plant proteins, animal proteins, human proteins – millions of them, all different – but all built up from the same 20 building blocks, the amino acids, in long chains. These can be arranged in any order and there may be several hundred amino acids in a single protein molecule. You can readily see how many proteins can be made when you think that there are 20 possible different amino acids in the first place of the chain, 20 in the second, 20 in the third and so on for perhaps 400 places. The number is $20 \times 20 \times 20$, 400 times. The number is unimaginably huge – there are over three million different ways of arranging amino acids in the first 5 places alone!

The amino acids themselves are relatively simple substances. If we start with acetic acid, the acid of vinegar, we can write its structural formula thus:

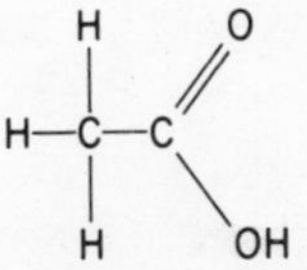

$$\begin{array}{ccc} H & & O \\ | & & \nearrow \\ H-C-C & & \\ | & & \searrow \\ H & & OH \end{array} \qquad \text{or } CH_3 . COOH$$

which you will recognize is the simplest of the fatty acid series.

To make an amino acid we replace a hydrogen atom, on the carbon next to the one with the $= O$ on it, with an amino acid group, $-NH_2$ (which is very closely related to ammonia, NH_3). Aminoacetic acid, also known as glycine, is thus:

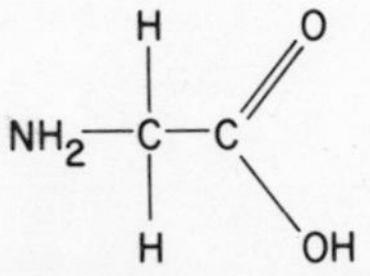

$$\begin{array}{ccc} H & & O \\ | & & \nearrow \\ NH_2-C-C & & \\ | & & \searrow \\ H & & OH \end{array} \qquad \text{or } CH_2NH_2 . COOH$$

Proprionic acid is the next fatty acid up the series from acetic acid. Its formula is $CH_3CH_2.COOH$. The corresponding amino acid, alanine, has the following structure:

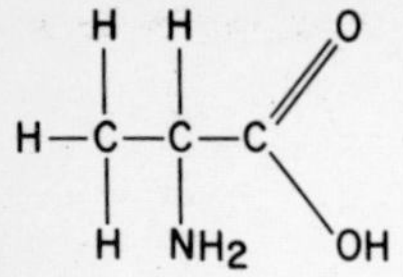

$$H-\underset{\underset{H}{|}}{\overset{\overset{H}{|}}{C}}-\underset{\underset{NH_2}{|}}{\overset{\overset{H}{|}}{C}}-C\overset{O}{\underset{OH}{\diagup}} \qquad \text{or } CH_3CH\,NH_2\,.COOH$$

The carbon with the $-NH_2$ group attached, known as the α-carbon and having four different chemical groups attached to it, may exist with them in two different spatial arrangements, which are the mirror image of each other. All amino acids in proteins exist in one of these arrangements only, the mirror images never being found naturally, though chemists can make them artificially.

The other amino acids will differ from alanine and glycine at the left-hand end of the molecules as they are shown above. The part $-CHNH_2.COOH$ is common to all of them. In glycine a hydrogen is added, in alanine CH_3 is added, and in the others, various short chains or rings of carbon atoms, with hydrogen, oxygen, sulphur or even further $-NH_2$ groups are also present. This end of the molecule is frequently given the single letter 'R', so the general formula for amino acids is $R.CHNH_2.COOH$.

When amino acids combine to form proteins, they do this through the NH_2 group of one amino acid reacting with the $COOH$ of another amino acid, splitting off water, $H:OH$, in the process. This link is known as a peptide link, and the proteins are known as polypeptides or peptide chains. A chain of amino acids may be written as:

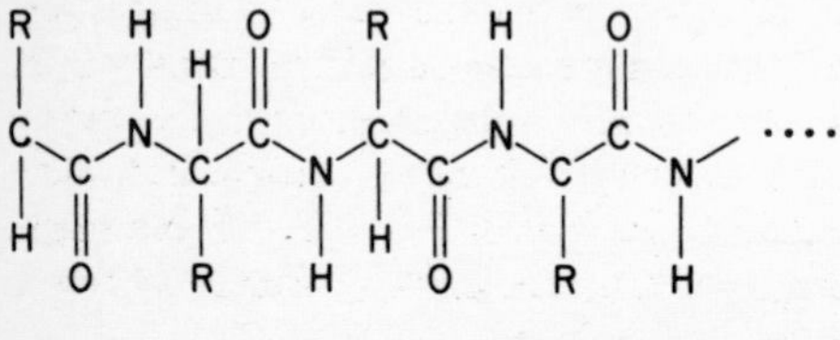

$$\begin{array}{c}\text{(peptide chain diagram)}\end{array}$$

When the whole thing is put together in three dimensions, the R side-chains have to fit together without colliding with each other. Side-chains consisting only of carbon and hydrogen tend to come together, for they shun water. Side-chains with oxygen or NH_2 groups will mix with water so these also occupy adjacent places when the peptide chain of a protein folds itself up, as it always will if it can.

Side-chains of some amino acids can be made in the body, but those of eight amino acids must be present in the diet, as must the NH_2 groups themselves. The eight essential acids are isoleucine, leucine, lysine, methionine, phenylalanine, threonine, tryptophan and valine. Histidine and taurine may be needed in children only. Not all proteins contain all the amino acids. This is of significance particularly with these eight amino acids. All are present in most proteins of animal origin, but protein from plant foods, especially those of seeds, are deficient in one or more amino acids. Thus grain proteins lack lysine, and pulse (beans, etc.) proteins are short of methionine. Foods from these two different sources can be selected that contain a balance of all essential amino acids. Most of such pairs contain a grain (cereal) material and one of the pulses, such as red kidney beans with tortilla in Mexico, dahl with chapati in India or even baked beans on toast in the United Kingdom. Animal connective tissue protein, collagen and its cooked derivative, gelatin, only contain a few amino acids, recurring many times in their chain molecules.

Digestion of proteins

Although the chemical links between adjacent amino acids are all the same peptide bonds, the side-chains of amino acids ensure that the immediate surroundings of the peptide bonds are all different. A single type of peptidase could not split up a protein chain into its constituent amino acids in the same way that a single glucosidase or lipase can split polysaccharides or fat into glucose or fatty acids respectively. Several different peptidases act on the proteins of our foods, each attacking peptide bonds adjacent to particular side-chains on the amino acids. Other enzymes attack each end of a peptide chain, lopping off single amino acids one after another.

The stomach secretes one enzyme, pepsin, that acts best in an acid medium. The pancreas secretes another three, trypsin, chymotrypsin and aminopeptidase. The first two of these, and also pepsin, attack peptide bonds adjacent to different specific amino acids, while aminopeptidase splits off amino acids from one end of the chain. In the borders of cells lining the small intestine are peptidases that attack the other end of the chain and pairs or short chain lengths of amino acids. Special types of protein, like the collagen and elastin of connective tissue have their specific collagenases and elastases to split up these molecules into their component amino acids, sugars and amino-sugar molecules. Most of the protein in the food is digested to single amino acids and absorbed as such. In infants, however, it is believed that whole antibody proteins secreted in the mother's milk may be absorbed from the gut, conferring protection against micro-organism infections. It is also possible that foreign proteins from cow's milk or wheat flour may, if given at this time of life, set up protective antibody production in the infant that occasionally may subsequently cause 'food intolerances' or 'food allergies'. Some vegetable food proteins are less completely digested than are animal proteins; as much as 20% of some lentil proteins may fail to be absorbed.

Protein metabolism

The amino acids all pass into the bloodstream from the intestines and so inevitably go to the liver. They pass (at any rate in part) into the cells of the liver, which enlarge. Nonetheless some pass on into the general circulation, for an increase of amino acids in the blood has been definitely proved to follow a protein meal. It has been shown that if these amino acids are not accompanied by glucose or fat, they are converted by enzymes in the liver into sources of energy. These enzymes (deaminases) remove the amino portion and change it into urea, which passes into the bloodstream and is excreted in the urine – in other words valuable amino acids are lost to the body. After the amino group is removed the residue is changed either to glucose or to fatty acid, according to the nature of the amino acid. Leucine, phenylalanine and tyrosine are changed to fatty acid and then to acetic acid; while alanine, glutamic acid and others are changed to glucose. The fatty acid and the glucose so formed are utilized as energy sources, as described in Chapters 4 and 5. About 60% of the protein follows the glucose path and the rest the fatty acid path.

Unless carbohydrate or fat accompanies protein intake, amino acids will not pass beyond the liver, but will be used as fuel for the body. When carbohydrate or fat intake accompanies protein it is supposed that they inhibit the action of the deaminases. The amino acids escape their action, pass into the general circulation and can be utilized for tissue-building purposes.

There is a continual interchange between the amino acids of the circulation and those of the tissues. Sometimes it is whole amino acids that are interchanged, sometimes it is the amino groups only, sometimes the rest of the amino acid or perhaps only its COOH group.

In any case there will be amino acids in the blood, whether they come from the food directly or arise from the tissues as a result of interchange. These slowly disappear from the blood, tackled by the deaminases in the liver and changed to urea which is excreted in the urine.

All the protein metabolism so far described is called *exogenous protein metabolism,* meaning the metabolism of amino acids that have arisen directly from the protein eaten. That, of course, is not the end of the story. Some of the amino acids circulating in the blood are used to build up internal secretions, e.g. adrenaline, thyroxine and insulin. These are oxidized or in some way got rid of after they have done their work. Some amino acids are used to manufacture creatine, essential in carbohydrate metabolism in muscle, and this substance in the form of creatinine is continually being lost to the body in the urine. Others are built into the protein enzymes and structures of the living cell. Still others are used to manufacture the nucleoproteins essential to the nuclei of cells.

What happens to these afterwards we cannot as yet completely determine. The internal secretions form such a minute part of the problem that it is scarcely worth while to follow them up. The creatine we can adequately measure, and its nitrogen forms a large part of the total nitrogen excreted during starvation. We cannot follow the history of the amino acids built into the protein of the cytoplasm except by means of isotopes, and what we learn suggests that when those amino acids leave the cytoplasm they are treated exactly as exogenous amino acids are treated. We can follow the amino acids built into nucleoprotein when, through wear and tear, they are discarded. The purine bodies, which are the nitrogenous hallmark of the nucleoproteins, are synthesized from such amino acids as arginine and histidine, but when the time comes for their rejection they pass by a path altogether different from that of their synthesis. They are transformed by the liver to uric acid and excreted by the kidney, usually as sodium urate.

All this intimate metabolism of protein digestion products that have entered into chemical and cytological structures we term *endogenous nitrogen metabolism* – i.e. metabolism of the nitrogenous substances arising from within the cells. We can trace it only in part, through creatinine and uric acid estimations in the urine.

Essential amino acids are needed in the various synthetic activities, as are the nonessential ones, the difference between them being that we cannot synthesize the former in our bodies. If they are not present in adequate amounts (one gram of each per day) in food proteins, then various body tissue proteins will be broken down to get at their content of essential amino acids. Skeletal muscle protein is the chief reserve that is used in this way.

The importance of these considerations is seen in their relation to high and low protein feeding. In high protein feeding the end results are predominantly of exogenous origin. The changes which go on in the liver in the conversion of amino acids to fatty acids, glucose and urea, involve a wastage of heat which cannot be used for any purpose except maintenance of body temperature. Because we wear clothes and live in warmed houses this excess of heat is not used for maintenance of temperature, but is almost sheer waste.

Reduced protein feeding will lead to tissue proteins being mobilized to provide the materials needed for various synthetic processes in the body. The turnover of amino acids may be raised and the total urea excretion raised, while tissue proteins, mainly those of muscles, waste away. This is seen to an extreme extent in untreated diabetes mellitus. Amino acids are then converted to glucose, which then cannot be oxidized and is excreted in large amounts in the urine, as is the urea formed from the amine nitrogen of the glucogenic amino acids. In fevers, burns, fractures and surgical trauma, especially when food intake is reduced, tissue protein amino acids are also used in the same way and a net loss of nitrogen occurs.

7

Other Elements in the Diet

So far, the nutrients that we have discussed have all been *organic* compounds, chemicals containing the elements carbon, hydrogen, oxygen and nitrogen. Most common proteins also contain sulphur in cysteine or methionine. Some, such as caseinogen, contain phosphorus and also have calcium attached to them. Phophorus is also present in nucleoproteins. Iron is attached to other proteins. In this chapter we will consider these and other chemicals or elements that appear in food analyses as *ash*. That is to say, these substances are left behind when the carbon, hydrogen and nitrogen have all been burnt away by excess oxygen.

They are commonly called the *minerals*. The amounts of these substances found in the human body, and in our foods, have an extraordinary range. An adult man may have over 1 kg of calcium in his body, whereas of chromium he has only 5 to 10 mg and of copper 150 mg. The amounts of some of these materials in the average adult are given in Table 7.1. The amounts of others, e.g. cobalt, silicon, tin, molybdenum, selenium and fluoride, present in the body are small, but there is evidence that their presence may be required. Cadmium, lead and mercury are three substances frequently present in our environment, including food, which are quite inessential in any amounts, but which are poisonous to living tissues, and will accumulate in them during life. Thus many adults may contain 20 to 30 mg of cadmium.

All the substances listed in Table 7.1 and those mentioned above as probably being required by a living body enter into the fluids, cells and other structures of the body and may be needed in definite amounts for the proper functioning of

Table 7.1 Average amounts of minerals found in the human body.

Calcium	1050 g
Phosphorus	700 g
Potassium	245 g
Sulphur	175 g
Chlorine	105 g
Sodium	105 g
Magnesium	35 g
Iron	2.8 g
Zinc	2.5 g
Manganese	210 mg
Copper	125 mg
Iodine	35 mg
Chromium	7.5 mg

these fluids, cells or structures. Thus sulphur is found in cell structures, contractile and other proteins, potassium in cell fluid and sodium in circulating and extracellular fluids. It is necessary to the functions of both cells and fluids that the potassium and sodium should stay where they are normally found, and in the normal amounts.

The minerals which are found in small amounts (less than 5 g) are probably working as catalysts or in a similar capacity. Except for the special cases picked out in the next section there is, so far, little evidence that we need to concern ourselves with these materials in diets for healthy people. Any substance to which we do not again refer is one about which no further significant information is known.

Important trace elements

Cobalt

Cobalt is a constituent part of a vitamin, cobalamin (B_{12}) which will be discussed in the next chapter. No other role is known for cobalt.

Copper

Copper is a component of many enzymes, and is required also for mobilization of iron from its stores as ferritin (of which more later). Children probably need 0.05 mg per kg body weight per day and the adult intake is probably 2 mg per day. Green vegetables, fish and liver are good sources. Milk is poor in copper and the liver of a pregnant mother loses copper to the fetus' liver to tide the newborn infant over the first few months of life. A prematurely born infant may not receive all of this copper and may thus become deficient. If copper accumulates in the body it is poisonous, especially to the liver and some parts of the brain. This happens if the liver fails to make a special copper transporting protein, caeruloplasmin. These patients can now be given D-penicillamine, which serves the same function, but the treatment must be continued for life.

Fluoride

Fluoride is essential for the production of hard, caries-resistant enamel in the teeth, but where present in water supplies at more than 2 to 3 mg/l it causes mottling of the enamel. At over 10 mg/l, calcification of ligaments and tendons may occur, leading to disability. A concentration of 1 mg/l water provides enough to so harden dental enamel as to halve the incidence of dental decay. The role of fluoride in dental health is discussed more fully in Chapter 16.

Iodine

Of the 25 to 50 mg of iodine in the body, 8 mg is found in the thyroid gland in the neck. In areas of the world where the soil and local produce are iodine-deficient, a great swelling of this gland, producing a *goitre*, occurs. This results because the thyroid gland incorporates iodine into its hormone, thyroxine, an essential metabolic regulator substance in the body. If iodine intake is small and not enough thyroxine is being formed, the thyroid gland is stimulated to grow. Probably somewhere between 150 and 300 μg iodine are needed daily in the food to enable an adult to make all the thyroxine needed. The amount obtained from all land plant and animal foods depends on geological chance – how much iodine the soil happens to contain. In the Mendip hills of Somerset, along the Cotswold and Pennine hills and in the Lake District of England soils are iodine poor, as they are in a wide area around the Great Lakes of N. America, and in the Austrian and Swiss Alps. Common table salt, can have the necessary minute amount of sodium iodide added to it by the manufacturer (such salt is sold in some British grocer's shops), or one can eat small amounts of any sea produce.

Although seafoods contain large amounts of iodine (herring has 200 μg/100 g), they do not make an important contribution to the usual diet. In Britain, milk and its products are the major source of iodine, providing 370 μg/dl milk in the winter and 700 μg/dl in the summer.

Manganese

Manganese is a component of some enzymes, but foods such as whole cereal grains or flour, pulses and leafy vegetables ensure such a rich food supply that deficiency has never been observed in man.

Molybdenum

Molybdenum may be concerned in iron metabolism and is certainly involved in the metabolic breakdown of nucleoprotein derivatives. Again, human deficiency has never been detected, for in the small amounts needed the diet is always more than adequate.

Selenium

Selenium-low soil associated with cardiomyopathy (failure of the heart muscle) was described first in the 1970s in China. Selenium is an element chemically related to sulphur, always abundant in human hair; both in China and in other regions where soils and crops are low in selenium content, low levels of selenium are present in hair also. Fish, both salt and fresh water varieties, can concentrate selenium and protect people in selenium-poor regions from the deficiency. The physiological importance of selenium is that it is a component of an enzyme that prevents the spontaneous oxidation of fatty acids in the body, which may result in producing highly toxic 'active radicals'. In this role vitamin E is also important (see Chapter 8).

Zinc

Zinc is a component of many enzymes essential for normal body function. It is closely involved with protein metabolism and increased amounts are required when protein synthesis is occurring, as in growth and tissue repair. In addition, tissue breakdown causes increased loss of zinc from the body.

The dietary intake of zinc is correlated with the protein content of the diet. Foods particularly rich in the mineral are meats and fish. Legumes and whole-grain cereals also provide zinc, although it is less well absorbed due to the presence of dietary fibre and phytate, which bind zinc and make it unavailable.

Leafy vegetables and fruit are poor sources of zinc. Average British diets may supply 10 to 15 mg zinc per day, although low-income diets are reported to be low in zinc.

Zinc deficiency may be associated with diarrhoea, apathy, loss of appetite, poor taste sense, peeling skin and hair loss. In adolescents, there may be delayed sexual maturation. Recently, it has been suggested that zinc deficiency may be a component in anorexia nervosa; treatment with zinc sulphate has been reported to restore normal eating behaviour in some cases.

Substances needed in more than trace amounts

Sodium and chloride

These have been put together because they so frequently occur together as common salt, sodium chloride, in the living body, in the cooking and eating of food, and in the physical world in sea water and rocks. In both physiology and nutrition it is the sodium that matters, for it is sodium that is actively transferred across cell membranes, from the gut, in the kidneys and between tissue fluids and all cells of the body, and it is on various sodium transfer mechanisms that regulatory mechanisms operate.

In fact the concentration of salt, the amount of sodium and chloride ions in body fluids, is quite critical for normal body function. It is important to consider the salt intake in the food and salt removal from the body in the urine and sweat. Normally, in temperate climates, so much salt is used in cooking and at the table, and so much is present naturally in our foodstuffs that the supply far exceeds the body's needs, and it is all excreted in the urine. Bacon, cheese, kippers, tinned meats, butter and margarine all contain salt to aid their preservation. Bread, biscuits and breakfast cereals all have salt or sodium bicarbonate added to them. In fact, it is difficult to avoid salt, as you would find if you had to prepare a low salt diet for anyone.

The body needs the salt to maintain the volume and osmotic pressure of tissue fluids and of the blood. Sodium aids carbon dioxide transport in the blood and the conduction of nerve impulses. In Addison's disease (a destruction of the adrenal gland), the kidneys lose their power of retaining sodium in the body, and many of the features of this disease are mimicked by a low salt regime, or by excessive loss of salt through the sweat in a hot climate or hot working conditions. Such a person is listless, mentally impaired, easily fatigued and pants vigorously on taking exercise. Muscular cramps may occur. The state may be seen in coal miners, steel workers, or in Europeans moving to a tropical environment. In Britain, the average intake of salt is 10 to 12 g per day, which is considerably more than the physiological need.

Excess salt accumulates in the body in some kidney diseases and in some diseases of the heart and the liver. Because of its osmotic effect, salt excess invariably leads to water accumulation and *oedema*.

It is becoming clear that dietary salt intake, perhaps linked with an inherited disorder in controlling salt levels in the body, is related to the development of a raised blood pressure. What is certain is that restricting salt intake to below 6 g per day, or giving drugs under medical supervision that encourage salt loss in the urine, are both effective ways of treating raised blood pressure in about 90% of people with this condition. Hypertension affects about 20% of people over 40 years old and is a major cause of other diseases of the circulation. We therefore need to attend to the salt content of food; the need to restrict this to what is strictly necessary on physiological grounds (replacing that lost in the sweat, etc.) is important in preventing the development of raised blood pressure and related diseases.

Potassium

This is found within the cells, but not in extracellular fluids. Thus muscle has 0.32% potassium while blood plasma has only 0.01%. When the kidneys reabsorb sodium into the blood they lose a little potassium, but the minimal daily potassium loss may approach zero. A normal diet contains about 3 g, and this amount is then lost in the urine daily.

There is some evidence that raising the potassium content of the diet relative to that of sodium prevents the development of raised blood pressure. Rich sources of potassium include fruit and vegetables, coffee, milk and some breakfast cereals. Processed foods, rich in sodium, are generally low in potassium.

Excessive losses of potassium may occur in diarrhoea or with some drugs, and potassium-rich foods may need to be taken. Only very rarely is it necessary to restrict a person's intake of potassium.

Sulphur

This enters the body as the sulphur-containing amino acids, methionine and cysteine. It is also present in the vitamin thiamine. The amino acids are required for protein synthesis and connective tissue materials, such as the chondroitin sulphate of cartilage. In a mixed diet there is little shortage of sulphur, as proteins from eggs, meat, milk and cereals all contain over 1% sulphur. Egg and milk proteins have 1.62 and 1.73% respectively, and this is largely as methionine. This amino acid is particularly important in tissue growth and regeneration after illness or injury.

Calcium and phosphorus

These two are considered together because they are both present in bone, in blood they have an important reciprocal relationship, and the high phosphorus content of some foods prevents calcium absorption. Both phosphorus and calcium have, though, many important roles in the body, independent of each other. Thus calcium is concerned with nerve impulse transmission, muscle contraction and blood clotting among its many important roles, while phosphorus is found in the molecules of the nucleic acids that transmit inheritance and build proteins, and it is intimately concerned with energy transfer and storage. In all living tissues phosphorus is present as *phosphate*, one phosphorus atom linked to four oxygen atoms and through them to metal ions such as sodium, potassium or calcium or to organic molecules, such as sugars, and purine or pyrimidine molecules in nucleic acids, for example. At the slightly alkaline state of tissue fluids or blood, calcium phosphate is not very soluble, so the concentration of each ion sets a limit to the concentration of the other and regulating mechanisms exist that ensure no unwanted deposition of calcium phosphate crystals in the body.

While there may be parts of the world where there is too little phosphorus in the soil or herbage for cattle, human dietary deficiency has rarely been described. All foods contain phosphorus (as phosphate), and dairy foods, fish and meat contain the most, followed by whole-grain cereals. However the outer layers of whole cereals contain phosphorus as phytic acid, which can reduce the absorption of minerals from the intestine.

Calcium enters the body in the food and some is inevitably lost each day in the faeces and in the urine. A balance exists in healthy and adequately fed people between the dietary intake and the losses. This is achieved by the regulatory actions of vitamin D and parathyroid hormone, which control the amount of calcium absorbed from the intestines, to match body needs. Thus, if bone growth is occurring (in childhood or in pregnancy), or if increased amounts of calcium are being lost from the body (in sweat or secreted in milk during lactation), then absorption will be increased to make more efficient use of dietary calcium.

In this way calcium balance can be achieved in a variety of physiological states, and on varying calcium intakes.

The amount of dietary calcium required to achieve balance has been and still is the subject of dispute and research. The DHSS recommended, in 1979, 500 mg for adult men and women, 700 mg for boys and girls during puberty, and 1200 mg for women in the last 3 months of pregnancy and while producing milk. However, a diet containing only 200 mg in Indian children still allowed the daily accumulation of 77 mg in their bodies.

In most other western countries, the recommended intake levels for calcium are higher than the British figures quoted here.

On a diet containing 1000 mg of calcium, 200 to 300 mg may be absorbed and the rest lost in the faeces. Once in the body this enters a pool, in blood and body fluids, of some 4 to 7 g. This pool is continuously exchanging calcium with the calcium of bone. There is over 1 kg of calcium in bone as calcium hydroxyapatite (formula $Ca_{10}(PO_4)_6(OH)_2$), and about 700 mg of calcium is daily removed from and added to this material. The urinary loss of calcium is withdrawn from the 4 to 7 gram pool in the blood, as are any losses in sweat or milk. The pool is maintained constant by two mechanisms. One is the action of hormones that control the rate of calcium deposition into and resorption from bone. The other is the action of a hormone that controls the rate of calcium absorption from the food in the gut. This hormone is liberated by the kidneys when the blood calcium concentration falls. The hormone is made in two stages by the liver and the kidneys from *cholecalciferol*, recognized for many years as vitamin D (see Chapter 8). The liver and the kidneys each add a *hydroxyl* (OH) group to the cholecalciferol molecule and the latter organs liberate it when more calcium is required.

The main dietary sources of calcium are milk and dairy products. In addition, cereals and cereal products may supply a reasonable amount of calcium, although this may be less well absorbed from whole-grain cereals due to the presence of dietary fibre and phytic acid.

Calcium may also be obtained from small fish in which the bones are eaten, dried figs, nuts (e.g. almonds and brazil nuts), parsley, watercress and black treacle. Unless these foods form a major part of the diet, their contribution to the total calcium intake will be small.

In parts of the world where the water is hard (i.e. contains many dissolved salts), it can supply a significant amount of calcium to the day's intake. In Britain this may average 70 mg per day, although greater amounts will be obtained in areas with the hardest water.

The sources of calcium in the British diet are further described in Chapter 10. In 1984, the average intake of calcium per head in Britain was 864 mg, and in all subgroups of the population considered by the National Food Survey, this represented more than the recommended intake level.

Various factors are known to promote or inhibit the absorption of calcium. Among the promoting factors the most important is vitamin D (in its active form), without which calcium absorption is negligible. The presence of active vitamin D in the intestinal environment depends on the body's need for calcium; it is therefore an essential promoter of calcium absorption when the need arises. Lactose (present in milk) also enhances calcium absorption by keeping it in a soluble form. Thus the presence of lactose, together with the large amounts of calcium present in milk, ensures efficient absorption of the mineral.

Calcium absorption is reduced by phytic acid present in whole cereals, due to the formation of insoluble calcium phytate. However, in the making of wholemeal bread some of the phytic acid is probably broken down during yeast fermentation. In addition, people who regularly eat foods containing phytate develop a phytate-splitting enzyme. Therefore, the overall inhibitory effect of phytate from wholegrain cereals on calcium absorption is not as profound as was once believed.

Oxalates, present mainly in spinach, may also inhibit calcium absorption due to the formation of insoluble calcium oxalate. Finally, some calcium may be bound by dietary fibre and lost in the faeces.

In the 1970s it was noted that there was a negative relationship between hardness of water and disease of the arteries of the heart. Where the water supply was hard, or richer in calcium salts, the incidence of coronary thrombosis and coronary artery disease was lower. As yet there is no explanation for this relationship. It is *not* here being suggested that a raised calcium intake directly protects the coronary arteries from disease processes.

In postmenopausal women and old men, the bones progressively lose mineral (calcium hydroxyapatite), become fragile and are easily broken. This is called *osteoporosis* and is discussed more fully in Chapter 13. At the menopause this is associated with the reduced hormone production by the ovaries, and may be prevented by hormone replacement therapy. However, the role of diet cannot be discounted and a high calcium intake prior to the menopause may minimize the effects of hormone withdrawal on the bones.

Magnesium

Of the 25 g magnesium in the body, about 5 g is present within the living cells, where it is mostly found in enzymes, particularly those associated with oxidation of foods and the transfer of energy. Like potassium, magnesium is lost from cells in states of chronic water and salt loss from the tissue fluids and blood, as in some longstanding intestinal disease with diarrhoea. It is also lost excessively in alcoholics. Normally about 300 mg is lost daily in the urine and, since we remain normally in balance, 300 mg is present in a normal diet. Most foods contain a useful amount of magnesium, since it is an essential component of chlorophyll in green plants, and is found in oxidation enzymes in animals. The foods low in magnesium are butter, cream, honey and white sugar. The phytate content of whole cereals etc. will prevent magnesium absorption just as it blocks calcium absorption.

Iron

Iron is part of the haemoglobin in blood, which accounts for two-thirds of the body's iron content. Blood haemoglobin concentration is therefore usually taken as an index of the amount of iron in the body. While the normal amount of haemoglobin in the blood is 14.5 g dl blood, the word 'normal' needs some explaining. For several years now, the incoming medical, dental and science students entering the physiology department at University College, Cardiff have had their blood haemoglobin measured. For the girls the average is normally between 14 and 14.5 g, but for the boys it is between 15.6 and 15.9 g. In other studies, other average values have been found. For sample populations drawn from both industrial and agricultural areas in South Wales the adult men had an average of 14.5 g and the menstruating women one of 12.5 g dl blood. It has always been thought that the lower figures for women are due to the continual loss of iron in the menstrual flow, that the resultant stimulus to haemoglobin formation is continually active, but that the haemoglobin content of the blood could never reach 14.5 g because of a shortage of iron. Medication with iron and all the other substances known to assist haemoglobin formation may raise the blood haemoglobin somewhat, but seldom to as high as the 'normal' male value. The stimulus to haemoglobin formation seems to 'switch off' at a lower point.

Iron is continually lost from the body in urine, sweat, and in shed epithelial cells from skin and gut. Altogether, in men, about 1 mg is lost daily. Women may lose 30 mg in the menstrual flow, so their loss averages over the months at about 2 mg/day. The iron needs of a normal pregnancy comprise: the iron content of the foetus (400 mg) and that of the placenta, uterus and blood loss at delivery (325 mg). This amounts to an iron requirement of some 2.8 mg/day.

The DHSS recommended intakes are given in Chapter 9 for adults and in Chapter 13 for children and adolescents. The average daily intake in Britain in 1984 was 11.1 mg per person, as found by the National Food Survey. However, for certain subgroups of the population, particularly large families and families with a low income, this level of intake fell below the recommended values. Further, a study in 1985 by the Ministry of Agriculture, Fisheries and Food of 15 to 25 year-old subjects found that the mean iron intake of all the women in this age group was only 8.7 mg per day, compared with a recommended amount of 12 mg per day.

This suggests that many people in Britain especially women and children, may be suffering from iron-deficiency anaemia. Alternatively, it is possible that the recommended allowance figures for iron are too high. This may indeed be the case in women who use the oral contraceptive pill, in whom menstrual losses are small, thereby reducing their iron requirements.

Why are the dietary requirements so much more than the daily losses? This is because much of the dietary iron is not available for absorption, and because the absorption mechanism is in some way sensitive to the state of the stored iron (ferritin) in the body. If the ferritin stores are full, dietary iron is rejected, and absorption only occurs when the stores are depleted.

In considering iron absorption, two distinct forms of dietary iron are identified. Organic iron, derived from haemoglobin and obtained from meat, is absorbed relatively easily, albeit slowly; the overall absorption of iron from meat may be 20 to 25%. Inorganic iron, present as iron salts mainly in plant foods, is poorly absorbed; absorption may be as little as 2 to 5%. In addition, it is profoundly influenced by other dietary factors.

Inorganic iron absorption is promoted particularly by the presence of vitamin C, which can increase absorption tenfold. This occurs due both to the reducing nature of the vitamin which converts iron to the absorbable (ferrous) form, and to its ability to keep this iron in a soluble state. Alcohol also enhances the absorption of inorganic iron in the diet. In addition, the presence of meat increases inorganic iron absorption.

Inhibitory factors include low stomach acidity, the presence of phosphates (including phytate), oxalates and tannin (from tea). All of these reduce the solubility of the iron, making it less available for absorption.

As a result of the interplay of these factors, the extent of iron absorption is difficult to predict. In addition, absorption is very dependent on the body's need for iron at the time. An average figures of 10% absorption is used in the UK. However, this may increase up to 70% in late pregnancy, when iron needs are high.

The dietary sources of iron are described in Chapter 10; they include cereals and their products, meat and vegetables.

Iron-deficiency anaemia is a widespread problem worldwide, affecting mainly young children and women of reproductive age. In many cases there are medical and economic reasons for the poor iron status.

Dietary iron-deficiency anaemia had almost disappeared in Britain during the 1960s and 70s. In the 1980s, owing to increasing impoverishment of poorer members of the community, iron-deficiency anaemia due to dietary iron deficiency has once again emerged in Britain.

As economic stringency returns to Britain, if all of the household's meat goes to the men and none to the women, as in previous generations, the women will increasingly become anaemic. This has implications both for their own health and that of any children they may have.

Acid-base equilibrium

The solid end-products of metabolism of a food may be either acidic or alkaline (basic). Thus meat, which is predominantly protein, gives acid end-products; fruits, even those that taste very acid, and vegetables almost all give basic end-products. Proteins contain sulphur and nucleoproteins also contain phosphorus. The sulphur is oxidized to sulphuric acid, while the phosphorus is already present as phosphoric acid, partly neutralized by organic oxidizable materials. These acids are neutralized in the body by basic materials such as sodium and potassium, forming neutral salts (sodium and potassium phosphate and sulphate). These reactions make blood and body fluids slightly more acid. This can only proceed a little way, for life is incompatible with a change of the blood from its normal alkaline state to neutrality (a pH shift from 7.42 to 6.97). The kidneys dispose of the non-gaseous acid substances, which is the cause of the acidic urine seen on a normal diet, rich in animal protein, or when fasting, even overnight. Why fruits, which taste acid, give rise to alkaline end-products needs some explanation. The acidity of fruit is due to organic oxidizable acids, like citric acid and malic acid. These are present partly as free acid and partly as potassium salts. The free acid and that partly neutralized by potassium are oxidized and the very weakly acid carbon dioxide is blown off in the lungs in the usual way. The potassium combines with some of the carbon dioxide, forming the weakly alkaline potassium bicarbonate. This makes the blood slightly alkaline and is excreted by the kidneys, producing a more strongly alkaline urine.

There is in all this an amusing double paradox. Foods which are neutral or even faintly alkaline (fresh meat or eggs) give rise to an acid urine whereas foods which are definitely acid to litmus produce an alkaline urine. Other acid-producing foods include whole cereals. Milk and all vegetables are alkali-producing, like the 'acid' fruit already mentioned. In any case, in the healthy *it doesn't matter at all whether one eats acid or alkali-producing foods*. The respiratory system and the kidneys are designed to cope with all the alterations in bodily acid/base balance that we can possibly induce by dietary means. As with the excretion of the nitrogenous waste products of protein metabolism, the kidneys cope with any excess of acid that even the high-protein diet of the Eskimo or Masai can give them. It is only when the kidneys lose their power to excrete acid due to chronic disease states that one needs to restrict the intake of acid-producing foods. The muddleheaded 'food reformers' who tell us to protect the kidneys by avoiding what they believe to be acid-producing, would restrict our intake of fruits such as oranges and lemons which turn the urine alkaline and, moreover, provide us with ascorbic acid.

8
Vitamins

Everywhere in the body we find catalysts acting on the host of chemical reactions that make up the function of living cells. While these are protein substances or enzymes, many require simpler compounds as 'cofactors'. Some of these latter are minerals such as calcium or iron, others are made freely in the body and are used to regulate metabolic processes, others again have to be provided in the food, for they cannot be made in the living body. Thus adrenaline and thyroxine are made in and secreted from the adrenal and thyroid glands and regulate various cellular reactions. For both, the amino acid tyrosine is needed, and thyroxine also contains iodine. Both of these, as we have already seen, must be supplied in the food.

The organic cofactors that we cannot make ourselves are termed the *vitamins*. Sometimes closely related materials, precursors to actual vitamins may be present in the food. They are called *provitamins*.

Vitamins were discovered late in the history of nutrition, for most are present in food in small amounts and their daily requirements are measured in milligrams or micrograms, not in grams. They are irregularly distributed in foods, belonging to no particular class of organic compound. Accurate and painstaking research was needed to identify their existence, to prepare the chemically pure substances, to find their chemical natures and to discover their metabolic functions. They were initially discovered by three converging lines of research: the study of diseases in people living on restricted diets, the discovery of similar diseases in animals, and the feeding of highly purified foodstuffs first to animals and then to people.

As an example we may take the disease beri-beri, in which nerve impulse conduction fails, leading to muscular paralysis and loss of sensation in the skin. The disease was found to be associated with a diet containing a great preponderance of white, polished rice. A Japanese admiral found it could be prevented by providing a more varied diet. Similarly, chickens or pigeons fed on a diet which caused beri-beri in man also developed a disease due to nerve impulse failure. This could be cured by adding to the diet some rice bran, or even a watery extract of rice bran. In Britain it was found that laboratory rats, fed on purified fats, proteins and carbohydrates and sources of inorganic materials, failed to grow and showed signs of muscular paralysis. These signs could be prevented if, to the artificial diet, a small amount of yeast extract, milk or swede juice were added. These three lines of work were brought together in 1912, simultaneously in Britain and Germany, and it was concluded that some essential food factor, not protein, fat, carbohydrate or mineral was present in very small amounts in rice bran, yeast, milk and swede juice. This substance was named provisionally *vitamine*, an amine essential to life. The name remains, but the terminal *e* is removed for many of the vitamins are not chemically amines.

It soon became clear that there was not one vitamin but several. One was present in fats and protected the eyes against disease, another was water-soluble, destroyed by heat and protected against paralysis, a third was present in citrus fruits and prevented scurvy. They were given letters of the alphabet, A, B and C respectively. A second fat-soluble material was then detected. It prevented rickets and was given the letter D. In the middle 1920s B was found to contain more than one substance, so it was divided into B_1 and B_2. By 1945 there were 10 known materials in the original B vitamin and two more were identified shortly after. Two further fat-soluble vitamins were detected in the 1930s and given the letters E and K.

Once the chemical structures and the functions of the various vitamins were identified, the letter system was replaced by chemical names which indicate the site of action, chemical nature or disease prevented by the vitamin. Vitamin A has become retinol; B_1, which prevented beri-beri, is called thiamine because it contains sulphur; while vitamin C is called ascorbic acid because it prevents scurvy, the Latin name for which is *scorbutes*. However, where there are several active forms of the vitamin, the original letter system is retained as a group name (e.g. vitamin E).

As well as knowing what diseases were prevented by which vitamins, it became essential to know how much of a vitamin any food contained. Before accurate chemical analysis became available, special units of activity were invented and internationally adopted in the 1930s by the League of Nations. *International units* were used to express the contents of some vitamins in foods, but actual weights – milligrams or micrograms per 100 gram portion of the food being considered – are now used. We may find that several related chemicals have the same vitamin activity, or are a third or half as active as the vitamin itself. In these cases the food composition tables speak of, for example, retinol (vitamin A) equivalent.

It is very fortunate that, for practical purposes, we do not have to pay attention to all the vitamins discovered. Those found first are the ones still most likely to be absent from a diet; and if the intake of these is satisfactory, it is most unlikely that we will go short of those more recently discovered. Exceptions exist to this, as to any other rule, and these will be mentioned in the following descriptions. In these, the fat-soluble vitamins are taken first, then vitamin C and finally the compounds originally included in vitamin B.

Retinol

This substance was originally known as vitamin A. Its ability to protect epithelia from infection endowed it with the name *anti-infective vitamin.*

In foods it is present either as the preformed vitamin or as a provitamin, many of which are found in vegetable foods. These provitamins are highly coloured and belong to the carotene group of vegetable dyes. *Carotene* takes its name from carrots, for it is the orange coloured material in these vegetables. It also occurs with chlorophyll in all green vegetables, though the chlorophyll masks the colour of carotene. Yellow-coloured fruits, such as peaches, apricots and oranges, and vegetables such as some sweet potatoes and pumpkins also owe their colour to carotene. Cryptoxanthine, the red colouring matter of Cape gooseberries and paprika also acts as a provitamin.

The provitamins are changed to retinol during absorption through the intestinal wall, about a third to half the provitamin molecule becoming retinol. The food tables quote both retinol content and provitamin (carotene) content, and the latter must be divided by 6 to obtain the equivalent retinol figure.

Absence of retinol or its provitamin from the diet over a period produces changes in the retina of the eyes, epithelial tissues, and in bone.

The retina is the light-sensitive cellular layer at the back of the eyes. It contains cells (rods) that are sensitive to dim light and this sensitivity is due to the substance *rhodopsin* in the rods. Rhodopsin (also called visual purple) is a compound of retinol and protein. Faint light splits the compound and initiates a series of changes that produce nerve impulses. Bright light completely destroys rhodopsin, the retinol being carried away in the blood. Rhodopsin is re-formed in the dark, but *only when* there is sufficient retinol in the blood. Retinol shortage, then, interferes with one's ability to see in the dark and this power is one of the most delicate ways of testing for retinol deficiency (though there are other forms of night blindness not due to this lack).

Epithelium is the name given to the cellular tissue lining the mouth, nose, trachea and bronchi, the digestive and genito-urinary tracts, the inside of eyelids and over the exposed part of the eyeballs, and to the glandular outgrowths of these various tracts and tubes. All epithelia depend upon a supply of retinol if they are to remain in good health and repel bacterial invasions. The epithelial coating of eyelids and eyes, the conjunctiva, together with that of the tear gland are particularly sensitive to retinol shortage, which produces dry, sore eyes, which readily develop bacterial conjunctivitis, xerophthalmia. Much of the blindness seen in children in poor countries is due to retinol deficiency, and such people also suffer from a low resistance to infection in respiratory and urogenital systems.

Bone, as we grow, is continually being reshaped, growing in one site and being resorbed in another site. Retinol appears essential for proper bone resorption, especially around the opening in the skull through which the cranial nerves pass. A late sign of retinol deficiency is pinching and degeneration of these nerves. Bone-forming cells (osteoblasts) are present in profusion, but there is a scarcity of bone-absorbing cells (osteoclasts).

The nature of retinol

For those who like to know chemical structural formulae, that of retinol is given here.

Since it is so largely composed of carbon and hydrogen, as are fatty substances, it is to be expected that it is soluble in fat and not in water. The one OH group at the end of the chain of carbon atoms puts retinol in the class of alcohols and enables it to combine with fatty acids and other substances. It can also be converted into aldehydes (retinal) and acids (retinoic acid).

It is a pale yellow oil, very easily oxidized when exposed to air and heat or ultraviolet light. Such oxidation destroys its biological activity. Ordinary cooking processes, however, do not harm retinol or the carotenes from which it can be formed. Cooking of, for example, carrots enhances their digestibility and so makes more of the carotene available for absorption.

The amounts recommended by the DHSS are given in Chapter 9 for adults and Chapter 13 for children and adolescents. They range from 300 μg per day for young children to 750 μg per day for adults. Needs do not increase in pregnancy, but an intake of 1200 μg per day is recommended in lactation.

Dietary sources of retinol are from animal foods; in particular these include liver, whole milk and butter. Margarine is fortified with retinol and is a rich source. Plant foods supply carotene; the major source of this is carrots, with small amounts provided by other vegetables and traces of carotenes in milk and its products. Overall, in the UK about two-thirds of the retinol equivalents are supplied by preformed retinol and one-third by carotenes. The total intake of 1377 μg retinol equivalents per person per day (National Food Survey, 1984) indicates that there is no problem with meeting vitamin A needs in Britain.

The contents per 100 g of some foods and fish oils are given in Table 8.1.

The human body can store considerable amounts of retinol (presumably in the liver), so an occasional meal of a food containing a large amount can redress several days of less than the recommended intake. In regions where the diet is deficient in the natural foods in this list, small amounts of fish liver oils, or liver from mammals can be used to make up the average daily requirement.

Acute poisoning may be induced by eating polar bear liver, but a more common chronic poisoning occurs when parents misguidedly dose their children with halibut liver oil as if it were cod liver oil. Daily doses of 30 000 to 150 000 μg (100 to 500 times the daily requirement) are needed to produce harm. Recovery is rapid following withdrawal of the doses.

Table 8.1 The retinol and cholecalciferol content of foods (μg per 100 g).

	Retinol equivalents	Cholecalciferol
Halibut liver oil	600 000–10 800 000	500–10 000
Cod liver oil	12 000–120 000	200–750
Polar bear liver oil	600 000	
Fresh herring	25–50	5–45
Tinned salmon and sardine	25–90	5–45
Milk	20–70	0.1
Cheese	360–520	0.3
Butter	720–1200	0.3–2.5
Fortified margarine	900	0.8
Eggs	300–340	1.3–1.5
Lamb liver	3000–30 000	0.5
Ox liver	3000–12 000	1.1
Carrots	600–1500	nil
Green leafy vegetables	?–1200	nil
Red or yellow yams	380–770	nil
White yams	50	nil
Apricots	70–280	nil
Bananas	10–30	nil

There is some recent evidence that a high level of vitamin A intake may in some way be protective against cancer. This is discussed further in Chapter 17. However, the possible hazards of excessive intake described above must be borne in mind. Similarly, vitamin A derivatives have been used in the treatment of acne and even to enhance tanning on exposure to sun. Again, care is needed to avoid overdosage.

Cholecalciferol

The second fat-soluble vitamin, originally called vitamin D, again has two provitamins, each of which can be converted into the active vitamin. The provitamins are sterol compounds, 7-dehydrocholesterol and ergosterol. The former is present in animal fats, including the oily secretions of sebaceous glands and the preening glands of birds. The latter is found in ergot, yeast and other fungi. The provitamins are converted into the active material by ultraviolet light. Therefore one could say that cholecalciferol is not a vitamin at all, since we do not need to take it by mouth. However, the sun does not always provide ultraviolet light, particularly between October and March in Britain or when our industrial activities add so much dust, smoke and water vapour to the air that the ultraviolet light cannot reach our skins. It is therefore important to remember that cholecalciferol present in food can replace that which cannot be formed in the skin in the absence of sunlight.

Once it is absorbed from skin or gut, cholecalciferol undergoes two further changes before it becomes active. In the liver an OH group is added at the end of the side chain, and in the kidneys, only when the blood level of calcium falls, a second OH group is added at the other end of the molecule. See Fig. 8.1 for the structural formulae of these compounds. This compound, 1,25-dihydroxycholecalciferol (1,25 DCC) then travels in the blood to the intestinal lining, where it potentiates the absorption of calcium from the food, provided calcium is available in the digestion mixture; 1,25 DCC also has a direct action on the kidneys, promoting the resorption of phosphate from the urine. Thus both the calcium and the phosphate concentration of blood are raised, a condition that favours the precipitation of calcium phosphate or hydroxyapatite, the crystalline component of bone.

Due to the existence of two sources of cholecalciferol, it has not been possible to determine accurately our daily requirement.

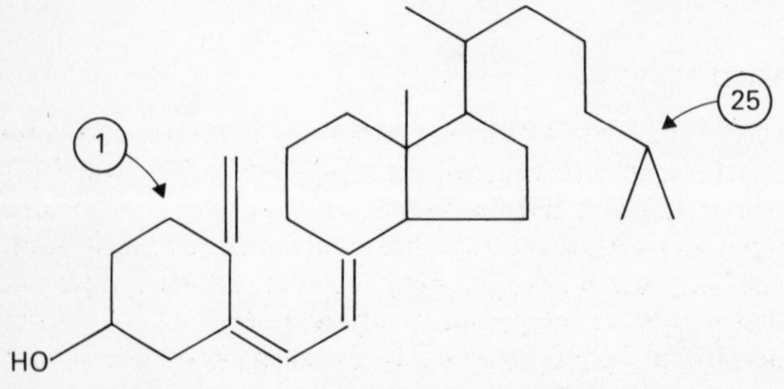

Fig. 8.1 The structural formula of cholecalciferol. The arrows indicate the positions where OH groups are added in the liver (C25) and the kidneys (C1).

The DHSS *Report 15* gives 10 μg per day as the recommended amount for individuals with inadequate exposure to sunlight. This might include the elderly, housebound and possibly some members of the ethnic minorities. For the majority of the population in Britain, sufficient cholecalciferol can be synthesized in the skin during the summer months, to meet the requirements throughout the winter.

The consequence of deficiency in children is rickets. The bones are poorly calcified and soft, so that limb bones bend under the body weight. The regions where active calcification *should* be occurring become swollen. In severe cases the blood calcium itself falls and abnormalities develop in nerve impulse conduction (tetany). A comparable disease, *osteomalacia* (literally 'softened bones'), is seen in adults.

The lack of vitamin D prevents the normal utilization of calcium. If in addition the supply of calcium is low, this may contribute to the picture seen in rickets. Thus rickets may be caused by lack of cholecalciferol and poor exposure to sunlight, coupled with calcium shortage. All three deficiencies will be accentuated by poverty in an urban environment and a temperate climate. The diet will be low in both calcium and cholecalciferol, industrial haze and climatic conditions will reduce sunlight. If one adds to these the presence of a dark skin and dietary restrictions and habits (such as extreme vegetarianism, for example), it is not surprising that rickets is still with us in Great Britain. The problem of rickets in the Asian immigrants to the UK is discussed further in Chapter 14.

Few foods contain vitamin D (see Table 8.1); it is mainly obtained from eggs, fatty fish, fortified margarine and some fortified foods such as breakfast cereals, yoghurts, bedtime drinks and infant foods. For the majority of the population in Britain the most consistent means of obtaining vitamin D is by skin synthesis on exposure to ultraviolet light. The day does not have to be sunny, nor the skin completely uncovered for synthesis to occur: light of the appropriate wavelength can penetrate thin cloud and light clothing. Sufficient time spent outside from March to October will ensure adequate vitamin status in the winter.

Occasionally children get too much cholecalciferol. This is usually due to parental mistakes. It causes a loss of appetite, thirst and increased urine output. The blood calcium may be raised, but it is not always, and abnormal deposits of calcium salts may occur. With removal of the cholecalciferol source, recovery occurs. A few children do develop high blood calcium on a normal cholecalciferol intake. The cause of this is not known, but they are best treated with a low calcium, cholecalciferol-free diet until their blood calcium level returns to normal and abnormal deposits of calcium salts have vanished.

Tocopherols (vitamin E)

These were discovered in 1923 and labelled vitamin E. They are fat-soluble materials found principally in seed oils, wheat germ oil having the most. Deficiency in rats causes sterility in males and abortion in females. Fatty degeneration and fibrosis also develop in muscles, a condition like human muscular dystrophy.

Vitamin E's role in the body is now being studied. It forms part of a system that protects the body (along with selenium) from highly toxic and reactive 'active radicals' that are formed by the spontaneous oxidation in the body of the polyunsaturated fatty acids, especially where these are present as components of nerve cell membranes and their myelin sheaths.

Since other reasonable sources of tocopherols include dairy produce, eggs and green vegetables, it is not likely that a person with a diet adequate for retinol and other major vitamins will ever suffer tocopherol shortage, so they can be ignored for practical purposes, whatever their protective role in the body.

However, since the transfer of vitamin E (as of other fat-soluble vitamins) across the placenta is generally poor, a prematurely born infant may be particularly vulnerable to vitamin E deficiency. This may be aggravated by the use of a formula milk which contains large amounts of polyunsaturated fatty acids.

Naphthoquinones (vitamin K)

These were discovered in 1934 in Denmark and called vitamin K because they were needed for clotting of blood ('koagulations vitamin'). These compounds are produced by bacteria, both in the human intestine and on plants. Approximately half of a person's daily requirement for this vitamin is met by bacterial synthesis in the large intestine. Problems may arise when the gut is made relatively sterile by antibiotic treatment.

Dietary sources of vitamin K include green leafy vegetables, liver and meat. Very small amounts are present in milk. For this reason, newborn babies may become deficient, and bleed spontaneously due to absence of clotting factors.

In adults, deficiency may be due to poor absorption from the intestine, or the liver, if severely diseased, may fail to use the absorbed vitamin K in making various clotting factors, for vitamin K is required in producing 4 of the 10 essential materials for blood clotting. Some similar materials can antagonize the actions of this vitamin, and so reduce the clotting tendency of blood. One of these, *warfarin*, is regularly used in medical treatment and also as a rat poison.

Absorption of fat-soluble vitamins

It should be mentioned here that absorption from the gut of all four of the fat-soluble vitamins is determined by the same factors that determine fat absorption. The bile salts aid fat absorption which, indeed, is grossly defective in their absence, as in biliary tract obstruction. Malabsorption syndrome, coeliac disease and sprue are all associated with defective fat absorption. Fat-soluble vitamin deficiencies may be part of the consequences of these disease states. Finally, some people take 'liquid paraffin' ('mineral oil' in the USA) as a laxative. This completely nondigestible material will dissolve the fat-soluble vitamins and so prevent their absorption from the intestine.

Ascorbic acid (vitamin C)

As early as 1601 it was known that oranges and lemons or fresh green vegetables could protect a person against scurvy, a disease that broke out after several weeks or months on a diet devoid of fresh or growing vegetable foods. The disease is characterized by bleeding into the gums which become painful, swollen and infected, bleeding under the skin and into joints which also become swollen and intensely painful. In 1747 a naval surgeon, James Lind, compared the curative effects of oranges with cider, hydrochloric acid, vinegar, sea water, and 'an electuary . . . made of garlic, mustard seed, *rad. raphan.*, balsam of Peru, and gum

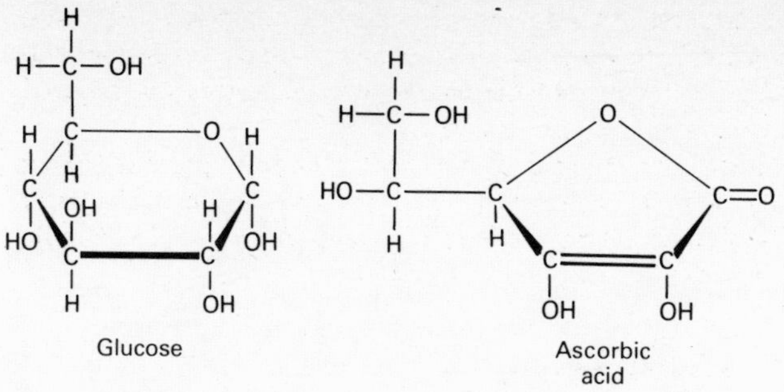

Fig. 8.2 The structural formulae of glucose and ascorbic acid.

myrrh'. Only those who had oranges recovered from the scurvy, which they did within a week. Despite this discovery and the gradual recognition by the British Navy that fresh fruit and vegetables were very important (hence the word 'limey') Captain Robert F. Scott was able to plan his expedition to the South Pole with no regard for prevention of scurvy. While the haemorrhagic state described above is the florid fully-developed disease, it begins with a swelling of hair follicles, filled with epithelial scales, and wound healing is delayed.

While ascorbic acid itself was first isolated in 1928, its identity with the anti-scorbutic vitamin was not shown until 1932. The chemical structure was soon determined and it can now be synthesized. It is closely related to the hexose sugars and its structure is shown in Fig. 8.2.

Ascorbic acid is a white, crystalline powder, very stable when dry, moderately stable in acid solution, but unstable in alkali. It is readily oxidized, initially to dehydroascorbic acid which also has vitamin activity. The two forms are inter-convertible, and are collectively referred to as 'vitamin C'. Further oxidation beyond dehydroascorbic acid causes loss of vitamin potency. Heat and oxidizing enzymes in vegetables both speed the process. However, heat destroys the enzymes and restriction of access of air prevents oxygen reaching the vitamin. These facts have implications on the way food preparation methods affect the food's vitamin C content.

In the body, vitamin C is present in small amounts in blood plasma and all tissues. It is concentrated in white blood cells and in the adrenal glands, and to a smaller extent in the liver and kidneys. Its major known metabolic role is in connective tissue formation, particularly after injuries, fractures or burns, when the blood concentration and urinary excretion both fall dramatically. In addition vitamin C is believed to be involved in the formation of some neurotransmitters in the brain, drug detoxification and iron metabolism in the body. It may also, along with selenium and vitamin E, exert a protective role in preventing the accumula-tion of 'active radicals' formed by the spontaneous oxidation of fatty acids in the body.

Measurements have found that there is a 'pool' of between 1.5 to 5 g of vitamin C in the body in an adequately fed individual. When this 'pool' shrinks to 300 mg, signs of scurvy begin to appear. It therefore must take several weeks of life on a diet virtually free of ascorbic acid before this limit is reached, though the time taken will depend upon the previous nutritional status of the individual. One thing that is clear from these studies is that filling the pool during one harvest season (for many fresh fruit contain an abundance of ascorbic acid) will enable one to survive for many months on a diet poor in ascorbic acid, though by the following spring, unless there is continual access to citrus fruit and fresh vegetables, the reserves may be depleted.

The availability in Britain of the potato as one of the staple foods ensures that outright scurvy is a very rare occurrence. This is because of a moderate, consistent intake of vitamin C from potatoes, eaten in their many forms. There is considerable variability in the recommended amount figures set by the various international authorities. Those set by the DHSS given in Chapter 9 (adults) and Chapter 13 (children and adolescents) are based on amounts of vitamin C sufficient to prevent scurvy. They are amongst the lowest figures recommended worldwide for vitamin C intake. Other authorities set figures that are designed to be 'optimal intakes', which may prevent marginal vitamin C deficiency.

It is possible that the elderly may be particularly at risk of such a marginal deficiency. In older people the absorption of vitamin C from the food becomes less efficient, so their dietary intake must be protected. Since old people spend more of their lives in institutions than the young, and they may have difficulty in eating some of the foods rich in vitamin C, they are definitely at risk of becoming deficient in this vitamin and their carers must take active steps to prevent this deficiency from developing.

While vitamin C is fairly widely distributed in fruits and vegetables, it is easily destroyed by various cooking and preserving processes.

Storage and marketing

It has been claimed that even a single day's lapse between harvesting and eating fresh fruits or vegetables significantly lowers their vitamin C content. This is almost certainly untrue. Wilting, bruising and exposure of cut surfaces to the air does decrease vitamin C. Storage of potatoes does lead to a slow progressive loss of their vitamin C, so that by March or April, only a quarter of the original content remains.

Preparation

In grating or fine shredding of fresh vegetables, e.g. cabbage, a considerable proportion of the vitamin C is lost, even in a few minutes. A very sharp knife, which reduces bruising, will minimize the loss.

Cooking

While heat destroys ascorbic acid, if given time, a temperature above 85°C also inactivates the oxidizing enzymes that themselves destroy the vitamin. So a short period of cooking, following a rapid rise in temperature may preserve much of the vitamin C of the fresh vegetables. The vitamin is dissolved out into the cooking water, so as little as possible should be used, and the vegetables cooked, as far as is convenient, in the steam above the boiling water. The water, ideally, should be brought to the boil and the freshly shredded vegetables added to it at such a rate that it does not cease boiling. A close-fitting lid should then cover the pan. For

200 g (about 2 medium servings) of chopped cabbage, 2 to 3 minutes of boiling is sufficient.

Addition of sodium bicarbonate greatly increases the destruction of vitamin C, and should be avoided.

Keeping vegetables hot for some time after cooking is very destructive of vitamin C. In 15 minutes a quarter of the original amount is lost, and after 90 minutes, three-quarters. In institutional catering the staff like to get through the cookery as early as possible and keep the cooked foods hot for servings over 1 or 2 hours. Vegetables served in a restaurant or canteen may have only a third of the ascorbic acid with which they started from the kitchen.

The problem is greater still where food is transported some distance from the kitchen for consumption. It is almost inevitable in this case that vegetables will be kept hot for a time and vitamin C loss will occur. This is a problem in institutional catering such as in hospitals, and fresh, raw vegetables should be served frequently to compensate.

Canning and bottling

Originally much loss was thought to be inevitable, but actual experimentation has shown that canned fruit or vegetables, even after prolonged storage, may actually contain more ascorbic acid than those bought on the open market and cooked at home. The reasons are: (a) none but the best quality material is preserved; (b) the time between picking, and preserving is shorter as it does not include marketing (wholesale and retail), and taking home and cooking, (c) the oxidizing enzymes are rapidly destroyed by the 'blanching' process when done on a large scale, and (d) the food is packed and preserved out of contact with oxygen. In these respects, the household bottling process may not be as successful as the industrialized methods. Very similar arguments apply to the large-scale deep-freezing of vegetables and fruit.

Vitamin C content of foods

As shown in Chapter 10, the major sources of this vitamin in the British diet are fruit and vegetables. The single most consistent source is potatoes, although their content per 100 g is not exceptionally high and falls on storage. The richest vegetables include brussel sprouts, broccoli, green peppers, tomatoes and bean sprouts. Among the fruit, citrus fruits and blackcurrants have the highest content per 100 g. Very little vitamin C is obtained from animal foods; milk provides a small contribution in Britain.

Despite the widespread distribution of vitamin C in fruit and vegetables, there are some groups of people whose intake of the vitamin may be precariously low. These include the poor, some elderly persons, people living in long-stay institutions and young people who exist on a convenience-food diet with no fresh fruit or vegetables.

This description of vitamin C cannot be completed without some mention of the supposed effects of large doses of the vitamin. While several separate, well-controlled sets of observations have shown that a well-fed person uses about 45 mg daily, and can remain healthy on as little as 10 mg, the studies that claim that 1 to 2 g daily promotes optimal health and prevents the development of the common cold have not been confirmed, and the claims rest upon very tenuous foundations. It is, moreover, possible that such large doses may actually be harmful, since they may affect bone metabolism and increase urinary oxalate excretion, with the danger of forming renal stones. Nutritional notions that are not backed by sound reasoning and experimental evidence should be ignored.

Thiamine

This substance is the original water-soluble, heat-labile vitamin B. It prevents the symptoms and signs of beri-beri and of similar diseases in animals. Its structural formula is shown below.

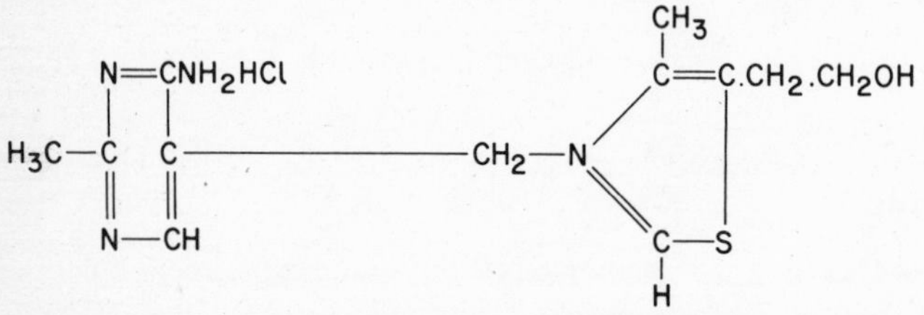

The left-hand ring of nitrogen and carbon atoms is one that turns up in many compounds in living tissues, including the nucleic acids, the carriers of genetic information. The right-hand ring, containing carbon, nitrogen and sulphur atoms, is but rarely found in living organisms other than in thiamine. The substance is an essential cofactor for one of the key enzymes in carbohydrate metabolism. It allows pyruvic acid, the product of nonoxidative breakdown of glucose, to enter the oxidation system, in which 90% of the energy of glucose is released.

Whenever a person eats a thiamine deficient diet he or she will develop beri-beri. Since in no diet is the vitamin totally absent, the onset of the disease is usually insidious. It starts with excessive fatigue, sensations of heaviness and stiffness in leg muscles, inability to walk far, and abnormal breathlessness on exercise. Sufferers may also complain of mental and mood changes, and later of sensory loss and abnormal sensations from the skin. When examined they may be anaemic, and the heart rate is abnormally fast on exercise. An excess of tissue fluid is seen in the legs – a sign of weakness of the heart muscle.

Since thiamine is so closely concerned in carbohydrate oxidation, it is not surprising that thiamine deficiency produces problems mainly related to the one tissue of the body, the nervous system, that uses carbohydrate oxidation almost exclusively as its source of energy, and that pyruvic acid should appear in the blood in sufferers from beri-beri or in thiamine-deficient animals. Thiamine requirements are also found to be related roughly to total energy turnover and to carbohydrate intake in the diet. In fact, a thiamine:energy ratio was accepted by a joint FAO/WHO committee in 1967. This ruled that for every MJ of energy in the food intake, there should be an intake of 96 μg thiamine, though the critical lower level of sufficiency might be around 60 μg thiamine per MJ of food energy. At this level 480 μg would cover basal energy requirements and 960 μg (0.96 mg) would be just enough for a very energetic person. If one accepts the internationally accepted ratio, this amount is the daily required intake for the normal sedentary person with a daily energy turnover of 10 MJ. The amounts needed for all ages and types of person can be calculated similarly from the accepted thiamine:energy ratio.

The important sources of thiamine in the UK diet are described in Chapter 10. Thiamine is found in cereals, pulses, pork and yeast; potatoes contribute a small amount of thiamine in the British diet.

The process of milling reduces the thiamine content of cereal grains, as much of the thiamine is found in the outer layers of the grain. Thus polished rice and 70% extraction wheat flour (used in white bread) are very low in thiamine. Wholemeal bread contains about three times as much thiamine as white bread made from unfortified flour. The thiamine added by UK government order to 70% extraction flour restores most of that lost in the milling process. In the cooking of rice, since thiamine is both soluble and heat-labile, considerable quantities of thiamine are lost, of that which parboiling before milling had preserved in the white-grain rice.

Thiamine deficiency has traditionally been found in poor, rice-eating communities, where the low thiamine content of the polished rice eaten was not supplemented from other foods in the diet. As the diet becomes more varied, so beri-beri decreases.

In the West, beri-beri is most likely to be seen in alcoholics, whose poor diet and increased metabolic need for thiamine make them especially vulnerable. Severe thiamine deficiency may develop affecting mental function or heart muscle activity.

Nicotinic acid

This substance was known to organic chemists in the nineteenth century, extracted from yeast and rice bran in the search for thiamine in 1913, but only finally identified as a vitamin in 1933. That a protein-free extract of meat or yeast prevented the human disease of pellagra was known by the middle 1920s, but in some way pellagra seemed to be *caused* by eating maize meal. Finally, by 1933, it was clear that the pellagra-preventing factor of meat or yeast was nicotinic acid or the closely related nicotinamide, that the vitamin could be made in the human body from the amino acid tryptophan (60 mg tryptophan producing 1 mg nicotinic acid), and we now know that the association of pellagra with maize is due to the absence of tryptophan in the maize protein, zein, and to its nicotinic acid being unabsorbable unless (as in Mexican tortilla making) the maize is treated with lime.

The structural formulae of nicotinic acid and of nicotinamide, the form in which it is found in the body, are as follows:

Nicotinic acid   Nicotinamide

Nicotinamide is a component of enzymes associated in all living beings with oxidative metabolism. Pellagra consists of inflammation in the skin and digestive tract (dermatitis and diarrhoea) and changes in the nervous system similar to beri-beri, though in pellagra these have been associated more with a generalized dementia (giving the '3Ds'). The earliest indications of the disease are redness of the skin in areas exposed to sunlight, and mental dullness. The disease is still common in many regions where maize is the main source of energy in the food. It is also found in certain parts of the world, such as India, where millets are eaten. These are high in lysine, which inhibits the use of tryptophan for nicotinic acid formation.

Nicotinic acid requirement is believed to be related to the *basal* energy needs of individuals. Thus, in the DHSS *Report 15*, the figures for recommended amounts are calculated on the basis of MJ of resting energy metabolism, rather than total energy expenditure as is the case with thiamine. The figures are given in Chapter 9 and 13.

In considering sources of nicotinic acid, it is necessary to take into account potential nicotinic acid, derived from tryptophan. Although this conversion is only at a rate of 60:1, it can make an important contribution in the diet. In food composition tables such as those of McCance and Widdowson used in the UK, this potential nicotinic acid is given in addition to the preformed vitamin. In this way, total nicotinic acid equivalent contents per 100 g of food can be calculated. Preformed nicotinic acid is provided by meat, cereals and vegetables (potatoes are a useful source); all of these, together with milk and its products, also provide potential nicotinic acid in the form of tryptophan. Nicotinic acid is added to white flour in the UK to replace that lost in milling. However in Britain the average nicotinic acid intake of 28.4 mg per head is well in excess of the recommended amounts for all groups. Thus a deficiency, in normal health, is unlikely.

Riboflavin

This vitamin was identified at about the same time as nicotinic acid, but as a growth-promoting substance, not as the essential material needed to prevent a specific disease. Like nicotinamide, riboflavin is a component of an enzyme associated with oxidative metabolism.

The structural formula of riboflavin is shown below:

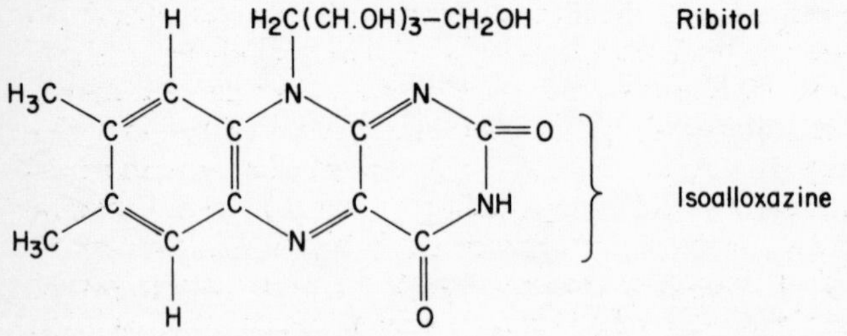

It is curious that despite the key role of this enzyme in metabolism, no deficiency disease comparable to beri-beri or pellagra develops in riboflavin deficiency. An inflammatory lesion develops at the angles of the mouth, and an appearance like that of chapped lips. Nasolabial seborrhoea also is associated with riboflavin deficiency. This is enlarged and blocked sebaceous glands on the nose, cheeks and forehead. In severe cases, capillary blood vessels invade the corneas of the eyes, with soreness and lacrimation.

As with nicotinic acid, the requirement for riboflavin is believed to be related to the *basal* energy needs of an individual. *Report 15* therefore calculates the recommended amount for riboflavin on the basis of MJ of resting metabolism. The figures are given in Chapters 9 and 13.

The major sources of riboflavin in the British diet, as described in Chapter 10, are milk and dairy products, meat (especially offal) and cereal products. Cereals themselves do not supply riboflavin to any extent, and it is only by the use of milk, eggs or specific fortification that cereal products become useful sources of riboflavin.

Milk is such an important contributor to riboflavin intake that it is often possible to predict a person's status of this vitamin from a record of milk intake. Some riboflavin may be obtained also from green vegetables.

Poor riboflavin status has been reported among some elderly people in Britain, as well as among adolescents consuming little milk or vegetables in other parts of the world.

Pyridoxine (vitamin B$_6$)

Three closely related compounds are grouped together under this heading. Their chemical formulae are given as:

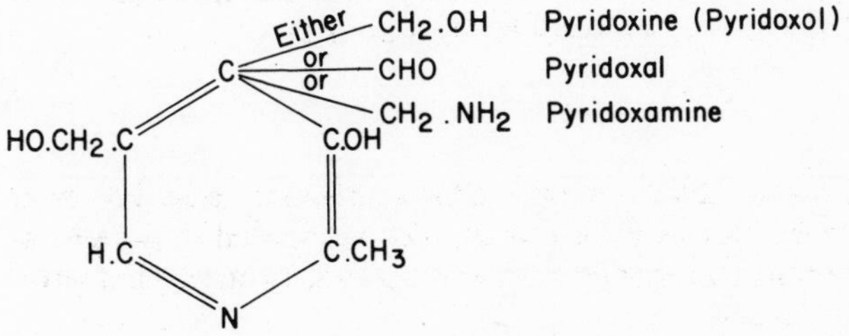

These materials are essential components of about 60 different (but related) enzyme systems involved in the metabolism of amino acids. The compounds are therefore widely distributed in foodstuffs and a purely dietary deficiency is very unusual. However, drugs such as isoniazid, widely used in treating tuberculosis, hormones and oral contraceptives all appear to increase the daily needs for the vitamin from around 2 mg per day to about 10 mg. Supplementation at this level reduces symptoms attributed to deficiency. Intakes greater than these confer no added advantage and may be dangerous. Recently, vitamin B$_6$ has been recommended for the relief of symptoms associated with the premenstrual period. Although there is no evidence for a deficiency, supplementation may help some women.

Cobalamin (vitamin B$_{12}$)

Although this substance was not isolated and its chemical structure determined until 1948–1955, its existence had been accepted since the early 1920s when it was found that protein and iron-free liver extracts could cure a form of anaemia called, because of its hitherto fatal outcome, *pernicious anaemia*. It is similar chemically to the iron-containing portion of the oxygen-carrying compound haemoglobin, but cobalt is the metal that occupies in this compound the place of the iron in haemoglobin. It is essential in forming nucleic acids and in maintaining the white insulating sheaths of nerve fibres. Its lack affects rapidly dividing cells, such as those of the blood-forming tissue and the gut, and also the nervous system. Red blood cells are formed in smaller numbers, those that are produced are large and more fragile, surviving a shorter time than normal in the blood – hence the anaemia. Vitamin B_{12} is synthesized by bacteria and the dietary sources of the vitamin for man are animal foods; these have accumulated vitamin B_{12} after its synthesis by bacteria within the animal's intestinal tract. Particularly rich sources are animal livers, where the vitamin is stored. Other animal foods, such as meat, eggs, milk and dairy products also provide vitamin B_{12}. Plant foods do not contain the vitamin; however it is possible that traces may be eaten arising from bacterial contamination of plant foods. The greater the degree of hygiene, the less likely this is to occur! Thus people existing on a wholly plant food diet (vegans) may need to take a vitamin B_{12} supplement (of bacterial/yeast origin) to prevent the development of a deficiency. Most vegans are aware of this need.

No recommended amount figures are given by the DHSS as the likelihood of a dietary deficiency in Britain is low. In 1987 the FAO/WHO recommended an intake of 1 μg/day as sufficient for adults.

A person who eats food containing 35 g animal protein each day will have the amounts of vitamin B_{12} shown in Table 8.2.

Table 8.2   The amount of cobalamin contained in the weight of food that supplies 35 g of animal protein.

	Weight g	Cobalamin μg
Cheese	138	2.75
Milk	1080	3.25
Eggs	260	1.80
Shin of beef (cooked)	115	3.60
Liver (ox, cooked)	120	105

Two very important points about this vitamin are, first, that it has to be combined with a substance produced by the stomach, *intrinsic factor*, before it can be absorbed and, second, that it is absorbed from the terminal part of the small intestine only. It is the absence of intrinsic factor, for reasons which are not yet fully understood, that results in a complete inability to absorb vitamin B_{12} and causes pernicious anaemia. This must be treated by B_{12} injections.

Where a dietary deficiency occurs due to a lack of the vitamin in the food eaten, the anaemia is simply described as a megaloblastic (meaning 'large cell') anaemia and can be treated by dietary means.

Removal of the terminal part of the small intestine as a result of disease, or in an attempt to produce weight loss in massive obesity, also removes the site of absorption for vitamin B_{12} and may ultimately result in a deficiency. The deficiency may not develop for some 3 or 4 years, however, as most people have stores of vitamin

B_{12} in the liver to maintain an adequate supply for the body's needs for this length of time.

The structural formula for cobalamin is very complex and will not be given here.

Folic acid

Anaemia that looks like pernicious anaemia, appearing in pregnant women, which responded not to a liver extract but to yeast preparations, was described a few years after the liver treatment was first discovered. By 1945 this factor, already shown to be present in many animal and vegetable foods (but only in small amounts in polished rice and 70% extraction wheat flour), was identified and called folic acid. Although it is now known to have numerous metabolic functions in the body, particularly in forming nucleic acids, the major effect of its deficiency is the development of anaemia, particularly in pregnant women. If this anaemia remains untreated, then a low-birth weight and possibly premature baby may be born.

It is also now thought that neural tube defects (spina bifida) may be related to poor folate status in the mother at the time of conception.

Folic acid contents of foods are difficult to measure; it is also not certain what are 'normal' levels for blood folate. For these reasons there is still debate about the requirements and recommended allowances for folic acid. None are given in the present DHSS *Report 15*. Figures produced by FAO/WHO in 1987 suggest 170 μg per day for adult women and 200 μg per day for adult men. These are lower than those previously published and reflect more accurate analytical techniques.

Major dietary sources of folate are green, leafy vegetables, offal and whole-grain cereals. Cooking, exposure of food to air and keeping food hot all lower the folate content of a meal. Reheating a meal two or three times can completely destroy its folate content.

The structural formula of folic acid is shown below.

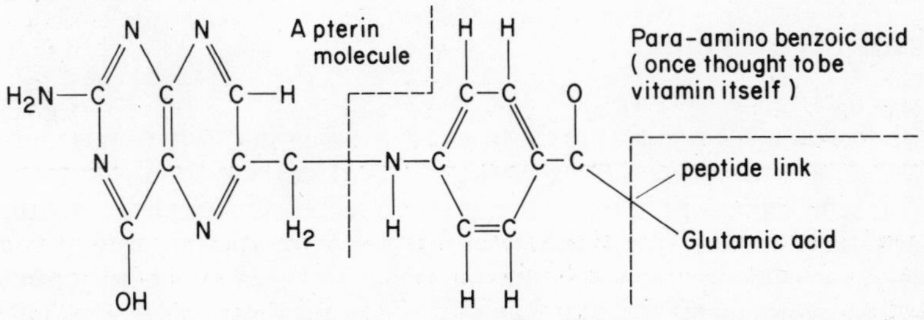

Folic acid intakes are correlated, in general, with income; families on a high income may have five or six times more folic acid in their diet than those on a low income. In addition there is a seasonal fluctuation in folic acid intakes, with lowest levels seen at the end of the winter, between February and April.

It has been reported that, in the UK, 20 to 25% of pregnant women exhibit megaloblastic anaemia related to folic acid deficiency. This suggests that in some sections of the British population, folate status is inadequate. In addition, the oral contraceptive pill interferes with folate absorption from the intestines, which may further lower folic acid status in some women.

9
Nutritional Requirements and Recommended Amounts

The preceding chapters discussed the functions of the nutrients in the body. The possible beneficial effects for health of above-normal amounts of certain nutrients, such as vitamin A and vitamin C, have also been mentioned; but what *are* the 'normal' amounts; how much of each particular nutrient does the body need to remain healthy?

The aim of this chapter is to identify these normal amounts, explain how they are derived and show how they may be used.

In practice the majority of people have no idea about the actual quantities of nutrients they require each day. Nevertheless, they generally stay healthy and meet their nutritional requirements by simply choosing a variety of foods, typical of their culture, which over the generations have ensured their survival in a healthy and fit state. Nutritionists, however, require more specific information on which to base scientific and reasonable advice. Two quantities are usually given for each nutrient: the minimum requirement, and the recommended amount. These are *not* the same, although they are often confused. It is important to recognize the difference between them, since they have rather different meanings and applications.

Minimum requirement

Each individual uses or loses a certain amount of every nutrient daily; this amount must therefore be made available to the tissues either from the daily diet, or from the body stores of that nutrient. If the nutrient is taken from body stores, it must be replaced at some later stage. Otherwise, the stores will become depleted and the person will be totally reliant on daily intake. If this is insufficient, eventually a deficiency state will develop. The amount of each nutrient used daily is its physiological requirement.

To decide on the numerical value of this requirement for any individual and any nutrient is very difficult. Firstly, an individual's needs are not necessarily the same from day to day. For example, more energy is used on a day spent shopping, playing sport and dancing, than on another day spent in bed, reading and watching television. Children exhibit considerable variations in activity, both between different children, and in the same child from day to day. In addition, there are daily needs both for maintenance of existing tissues and for growth, so that allowances must be made for this. The same applies for pregnant or lactating women, when additional allowances must be made for the nutrients needed for the development of the baby, and those secreted in the milk.

One solution is to look at the average requirements of groups of similar people and to define a reasonable minimum level. The age of the child is taken as a basis for defining 'similar' children; for pregnant women, the stage of pregnancy is taken as the common basis. If the intake of the particular nutrient falls below this minimum level, a deficiency is the likely outcome.

Another approach is to find how much of a nutrient the body is using each day. For this, all possible routes for the excretion of a nutrient or of its by-products must be taken into account. The amounts to be replaced can then be determined. This technique can however only be applied to nutrients that are excreted. Other nutrients may not normally be excreted from the body, and different measurements then have to be made. These may include measurement of blood levels, use of radioactive isotopes to measure turnover of the nutrient in the whole body, or determination of the amounts needed to reverse a deficiency state. The use of expired gas measurements and of heat output to determine the energy expenditure of the body (described in Chapter 3) forms the basis for energy requirement figures.

Even using all these techniques, there are still some nutrients for which it is difficult to make experimental measurements of physiological requirement. These include calcium, vitamin D and nutrients of which there are large reserves in the body, such as vitamins A and B_{12}. In these cases figures for minimum requirements are based on observations of actual intakes in populations that are healthy, and are therefore apparently satisfying their physiological requirements.

Finally, there are some nutrients, such as sodium, magnesium, vitamins E and K and many of the trace elements, where a minimum requirement has not yet been established, as these nutrients are so widespread in foods that it would be extremely unusual to eat a diet providing less than the minimum requirement, and so deficiencies very rarely occur in healthy people. Only where there is some disease, an unusual need for the nutrient, or an inability to absorb it, is a deficiency of these possible. However, these situations are not taken into account in the requirement figures, which are designed for healthy people.

Distribution of minimum requirements in a population

When measurements of minimum requirement are made in a sufficiently large group of people, the results usually follow a typical 'normal' distribution curve, as shown in Fig. 9.1.

This shows that the majority of people have a minimum requirement around the mean for the whole group — but some have a higher requirement and some a lower one. If the group is sufficiently large, then half of the sample will have requirements above the mean, and half below it. This is simply a reflection of what is meant by the term 'mean'; it is not something peculiar to nutrition, or requirements alone.

Practical implications

Having described how a minimum requirement distribution curve might be obtained, it is fairly easy to see one of its major limitations. This may be illustrated by the following example.

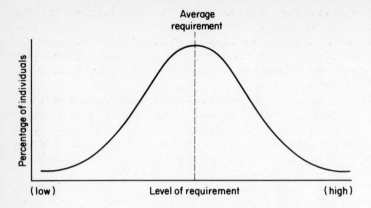

Fig. 9.1   The normal distribution of nutrient requirements in a population.

In a study of the energy intakes of 3-year-old boys, the curve shown in Fig. 9.2 was obtained. Three boys were found to have intakes of *a*, *b* and *c* kJ respectively. The following conclusions can be drawn from the results:

(1)   With an intake of *a* kJ, we can be fairly sure that this boy is not reaching his requirement for energy. He should be investigated further.

(2)   This boy's energy intake of *b* kJ is well below the mean for his group. However, this does not necessarily imply that he is receiving inadequate energy for his needs. He may simply be a child with a relatively low requirement. On the other hand, if in addition he is not growing normally, or is showing other signs of insufficient intake, his needs for energy and other nutrients are probably not being met, and his food intake should be increased.

(3)   At first sight the boy obtaining *c* kJ seems to have a more than adequate energy intake; it is most probable that this is indeed the case. However, the possibility does exist that he is a child who has a very high requirement and it may not be

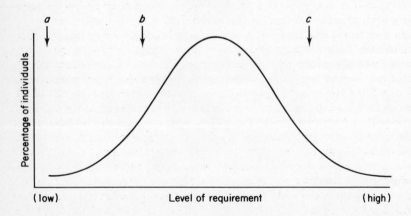

Fig. 9.2   Distribution of energy intakes in a hypothetical population of 3-year-old boys.

met by his present intake, even though it appears high. Therefore we cannot assume that he must be meeting his requirement.

Thus, a firm statement about the adequacy of an individual diet may not be possible on the basis of a population's mean requirement. It is only if an individual intake falls outside the range of requirements that a definite conclusion can be drawn about the adequacy.

In practice, it is the mean of the minimum requirements that is quoted for a group of people. This can be misleading if the reader is unaware of its derivation or meaning. It must be remembered that this figure is the mean of a range, and that almost half of the group will actually need more than this figure for the particular nutrient, and almost half will need less. A small part of the group will actually fall at the mean value, and require the amount given as the mean.

A more useful concept is that of recommended amount. Tables of recommended amount values derived from minimum requirements are published by government committees for use within their own countries.

Recommended amounts

The recommended amount of a nutrient is a figure which indicates the amount of a given nutrient that should satisfy the nutritional needs of all or nearly all of a healthy group of people. In general, the figure for a recommended amount is set towards the upper end of the minimum requirement distribution, so that the intake will be adequate for most people (usually 97%). It may be calculated roughly by adding 20% to the mean requirement figure. In this way, there is a high probability that the needs of the majority will be met.

A major exception to this is the recommended amount for energy. It is not desirable for people to eat more than their individual requirement for energy. Some of the dangers associated with obesity were highlighted in Chapter 3. Therefore the figures given for the recommended amounts for energy are the average requirements for the particular population group. In practice, some people will require more than this, and some will require less; the energy figures cannot be used rigorously to prescribe or evaluate one person's energy intake. They are however useful when the total energy intake of a group of people is compared against the calculated average recommendation for that group.

A further aspect which has to be considered when figures are translated from 'requirements' into 'recommended amounts', is the availability of the nutrient in food, and its degree of absorption from the digestive tract. It has to be remembered that the requirement is the actual amount of the nutrient which the tissues require each day. If the absorption of a particular nutrient from food is only 10% of that ingested, then it will be necessary to eat 10 times the requirement to ensure a sufficient supply to the tissues. Unfortunately, the absorption of nutrients from food is rarely so accurately predictable. Many factors promote or inhibit absorption. These interact, so the content of the actual meal eaten will determine what proportion of a nutrient is actually absorbed. In addition, there may be individual variability in the handling of nutrients by the digestive tract, carriers in the blood, or the tissues themselves. As a result, the recommended amount figure may include a percentage factor to compensate for these variables, making it considerably greater than the actual physiological need.

Table 9.1 Recommended daily amounts of food energy and some nutrients for adults in the UK. From: DHSS (1979). *Report 15: Recommended amounts of Food Energy and Nutrients for Groups of People in the United Kingdom.* London: HMSO.

Age (years)	Occupational category	Energy (MJ)	Protein (g)	Thiamine (mg)	Riboflavin (mg)	Nicotinic acid (mg)	Ascorbic acid (mg)	Vitamin A (µg)	Vitamin D (µg)	Calcium (mg)	Iron (mg)
Men											
18–34	Sedentary	10.5	63	1.0	1.6	18	30	750	a	500	10
	Moderately active	12.0	72	1.2	1.6	18	30	750	a	500	10
	Very active	14.0	84	1.3	1.6	18	30	750	a	500	10
35–64	Sedentary	10.0	60	1.0	1.6	18	30	750	a	500	10
	Moderately active	11.5	69	1.1	1.6	18	30	750	a	500	10
	Very active	14.0	84	1.3	1.6	18	30	750	a	500	10
65–74	Sedentary	10.0	60	1.0	1.6	18	30	750	a	500	10
75+	Sedentary	9.0	54	0.9	1.6	18	30	750	a	500	10
Women											
18–54	Most occupation	9.0	54	0.9	1.3	15	30	750	a	500	12b
	Very active	10.5	62	1.0	1.3	15	30	750	a	500	12
	Pregnancy	10.0	60	1.0	1.6	18	60	750	10	1200	13
	Lactation	11.5	69	1.1	1.8	21	60	1200	10	1200	15
55–74	Sedentary	8.0	47	0.8	1.3	15	30	750	a	500	10
75+	Sedentary	7.0	42	0.7	1.3	15	30	750	a	500	10

a = Adults with inadequate exposure to sunlight may need a supplement of 10 µg per day.
b = This intake of iron may not be sufficient for 10% of women with heavy menstrual losses.

The tables currently in use in the United Kingdom are those published in 1979 as *Report 15* by the DHSS, and are summarized in Table 9.1. Figures are given here for adults; those applying to children and adolescents are found in Table 13.3. on p. 151.

If the United Kingdom tables are compared with those produced by the Food and Agriculture Organization/World Health Organization (FAO/WHO) or by individual countries, differences both in the range of nutrients listed and the amounts recommended are found. This implies two things. Firstly, there are differences in needs between certain countries, as a result of differing life styles, so that when 'recommended amounts' tables are used, they should always be the ones relating to the country in question.

Secondly, opinions differ between the committees that draw up the tables in different countries as to the safety margins which should be added to the figures. As a result, final figures also differ. This does not mean that some are more 'correct' than others; it reflects fundamental differences in emphasis and serves to underline the uncertainty of recommended amount values.

It is important to remember that these figures are never an 'absolute' when considering their uses. They are basically a mixture of physiological and nutritional knowledge, human opinions and political/economic expediencies of many kinds.

The use of 'recommended amount' tables

Report 15 published by the DHSS in 1979, which gives the current recommended amounts for the United Kingdom, states that the figures should be used for:

(1) The planning of food supplies.
(2) The interpretation of surveys of food supplies, so that differences between groups of individuals and trends in time can be described.
(3) Drawing attention in surveys of food intake to subgroups that may be at risk. These may then be investigated further by other means.

It is important to remember that recommended amount figures should not be used to judge individual nutritional intakes for their adequacy (for which they are often used). They also do not cover any additional needs as a result of disease – they are meant for healthy people. In addition, the figures refer to the actual amounts of nutrients eaten; wastage is not included and allowances should therefore be made in meal planning.

It is very important for anyone involved in practical nutrition to be fully aware of these limitations relating to the use of recommended allowance tables. Frequently, they are used for purposes for which they were not intended, in particular for judging individual nutritional status on the basis of nutrient intake.

Although this consideration of recommended amounts has centred on the DHSS figures, issued for use in the United Kingdom, similar principles apply for all recommended intake tables published around the world.

10

The British Diet – What Does It Contain?

The recommended amounts for nutrients are set at the upper limit of the needs of the majority of people. It can therefore be assumed that if foods are eaten which contain the amounts of nutrients recommended, there should be no danger of nutritional deficiency; but which foods, or mixtures of foods, will actually provide these correct amounts? This question is considered in this chapter.

There are two approaches:

(1) *Tables of food composition*, available for indigenous foods in most countries, provide an analysis of the nutrients in each food. In the United Kingdom, the tables used are those of McCance and Widdowson in *The Composition of Foods*, currently in its 4th edition. Updating supplements are produced at intervals as information about new foods becomes available.

Using the information provided by the tables, a range of foods can be selected that when added together to form a day's meals will provide the recommended amounts of the various nutrients.

Clearly, this is an extremely laborious way of looking at the diet for the majority of healthy people. It must however be done if someone, for reasons of health, requires a very specific level of one or more nutrients in the diet. Then the amounts of food have to be very carefully calculated, as any deviations from the prescribed intake may have serious consequences. Calculations of this nature are done by dietitians, who tailor the diet precisely to a patient's need. For the rest, a much simpler approach is possible.

(2) In practice, it is not actually necessary to have a detailed knowledge of all the nutrients contained in a food. All that is required is to know what nutrients are present in the largest amounts and can make a significant contribution to the diet. Another factor determining total nutrient intake concerns the frequency of ingestion. Foods containing even relatively high concentrations of a particular nutrient contribute little to the average intake if they are eaten only once or twice a year. On the other hand, a food which has only a moderate content of say, vitamin C, will make a substantial contribution to overall vitamin C intakes if it is eaten daily, as is the case with potatoes in the British diet.

To identify the foods which are important sources of particular nutrients, both their nutrient composition and their frequency in the diet must be known. This information can be obtained from the National Food Survey report, which is published annually by the Ministry of Agriculture, Fisheries and Food in the United Kingdom. Other countries publish similar reports, and comparative studies may be made, for example throughout the European Economic Community (EEC).

The National Food Survey records household food consumption throughout the year, in a random sample of some 7000 households in the United Kingdom, selected to be representative of the population. From the results it obtains, it is able to show which foods, or groups of foods, were the main sources of different nutrients in the sampled population in any particular year. The food groups designated by the National Food Survey are based on common biological origins rather than on the nutritional functions of the foods. Thus they reflect more accurately the way ordinary people think of foods, rather than the more scientific approach of a nutritionist, who considers their nutritional content. The tables reflect both the importance of different food groups, and the nutritional contribution made by them to the British diet during the particular year studied. Since the study is done each year, it is possible to monitor trends and changes in food intakes in this way. Relative stability of the results from year to year suggests that the survey is in fact representing the typical UK eating patterns.

In view of this, the National Food Survey results have been used here as a basis for the consideration of nutrients in food. This is a more practical and useful approach than the traditional division of foods into groups according to whether they supply mainly energy, protein or whatever. It provides a more comprehensive view of the nutritional content of groups of foods and their place in our diet.

Table 10.1 summarizes the information from the National Food Survey published in 1986; it shows the contribution made (as a percentage) by the food groups used in the survey to the total intake of individual nutrients. It also highlights which nutrients are provided most particularly by different groups of foods. This information is repeated in bar chart form in the following sections.

Milk, cream and cheese

From Fig. 10.1, it can be seen that this group provides a wide range of nutrients, in important amounts.

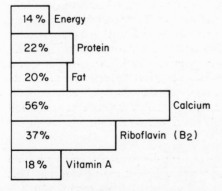

Fig. 10.1 Nutrients provided by dairy products (milk, cream and cheese) as a percentage of total diet (see Table 10.1).

Table 10.1 Contributions made by groups of foods to the nutritional value of household food (per person per day). Values are expressed as a percentage of the total diet. Note that values below 0.5% have been omitted. From: Ministry of Agriculture, Fisheries and Food (1986). *Household Food Consumption and Expenditure Survey.* London: HMSO.

	Energy	Protein	Fat	CHO	Calcium	Iron	B_1	B_2	Nic.a.	Vit. C	Vit. A	Vit. D
Milk, cream and cheese	14	22	20	8	56	3	11	37	14	5	18	9
Total meat	16	31	25	2	3	21	14	18	34	2	37	1
Total fish	1	5	1	0	2	2	1	—	4	—	0	14
Eggs	2	4	3	—	2	4	1	6	3	0	3	12
Total fats	15	0	36	0	1	1	—	—	0	1	18	52
Sugar and preserves	8	—	—	18	0	1	—	—	—	1	—	—
Total vegetables	9	9	2	15	7	18	17	8	15	50	22	0
Total fruit	3	1	1	5	2	4	4	2	2	40	1	—
Total cereals	30	25	11	49	25	42	50	20	21	1	0	11
Total beverages	0	1	0	0	1	1	1	4	4	—	0	1

Energy

Milk, cream and cheese provide 14% of total energy intake (of which almost 10% comes from milk alone). This group, together with meats and fats, lies joint second after cereals in importance as a source of energy.

This relatively important contribution to energy intake may be surprising, as milk in particular is not viewed as a high-energy food. It is a very dilute food, containing 88% water. Yet as a result of its frequent consumption, the energy it provides amounts to 10% of total energy consumed. Approximately half of this energy comes from the fat contained in milk, and the remainder from carbohydrate (lactose) and protein.

In the United Kingdom, relatively large amounts of milk are consumed. It must be remembered that in other countries, where the dairy industry is less important, the importance of milk as an energy source will be less.

Protein

Many people consider milk to be an important source of protein: this is substantiated by the Survey, which shows this group provides 22% of total protein eaten (14% comes from milk alone and 6% from cheese). As described for energy, the size of the contribution derives more from the volume of milk consumed, than from its protein concentration. Conversely the amount of cheese eaten is small, but because of the greater concentration of the milk protein, it provides an important amount.

Fat

This group of foods provides an important amount of fat (20%), lying third after fats and meats. Milk fat is unusual among the fats in the diet, in that it contains a high proportion of short-chain fatty acids, particularly butyric acid. This contributes to the characteristic smell of milk that has 'gone off'. The fat in milk is gradually being reduced in the UK as more dairies are making semi-skimmed and skimmed milk available for doorstep delivery. In a few years' time, the contribution to total fat made by milk may well be less.

Many cheeses still retain a large proportion of the fat in whole milk ('full-fat' cheeses), and some may have extra fat added. In this way they contribute markedly to the total fat provided by this group. In addition to lower-fat milks, there are also some lower-fat cheeses being made; again, these may have an impact in the future on the total contribution to fat made by this group. We have been used to seeing 'cottage' cheese for some years, but lower-fat hard cheeses are a relatively new item in the UK.

Calcium

The figure for the amount of calcium (56%) provided by milk, cream and cheese, is the highest of any of the contributions made by this group. This emphasizes the importance of milk and cheese during periods of growth, as it is then relatively easy to meet the high calcium needs. However, it is also important to bear in mind that although they are a very useful source of calcium, these foods are not irreplaceable. On the other hand, a diet which excludes all milk and dairy products does tend to be much lower in calcium than one including these foods. It is quite diffi-cult to exceed an intake of 300 mg of calcium per day without any dairy produce in the diet.

B vitamins

Milk, cream and cheese supply thiamine, riboflavin and nicotinic acid (made from tryptophan by the body), but only the contribution of riboflavin is particularly high (37%); this food group is the most important single supplier of this vitamin in the British diet. A potential problem is that milk left on a sunny doorstep, or exposed to light in a supermarket, does gradually lose some of its riboflavin. This is because the vitamin is unstable in light and is progressively broken down on exposure.

Vitamin A

Almost 20% of the total vitamin A in the British household diet is obtained from this group. This is largely as preformed retinol, although a small proportion is present as carotene. The amount varies between summer and winter, with the higher values occurring in the summer months. The figures given here are the averages for the whole year.

Other nutrients

None of the many other nutrients provided by milk, cream and cheese make a very great contribution to the total nutrient intake of British households. Reference may be made to *The Composition of Foods* tables for further information on these.

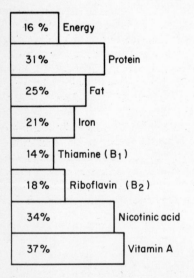

Fig. 10.2 Nutrients provided by meats as a percentage of total diet (see Table 10.1).

Total meat

All types of fresh, frozen, prepared and processed meats are considered in this section, as well as offal such as liver. The nutrients present in important amounts, from Fig. 10.2, can be seen to be energy, protein, fat, iron, B vitamins and vitamin A.

Energy

The meat group as a whole supplies 16% of the total energy eaten in British households. This is very similar to the energy provided by the dairy products and fats groups.

About 70% of the energy in meats is derived from the fat content and the remainder from the protein. Meat contains virtually no carbohydrate, as any glycogen that it originally contained is broken down after slaughter. Breakdown of glycogen is an important stage in the tenderizing of meat. A piece of meat that is relatively fatty will therefore contain more energy than one that is lean. It must be remembered that fat is not just present as the visible layers around the outer edges of meat. Quite a large amount is found amongst the meat fibres themselves and is therefore difficult to see and assess. In addition, many made-up meat products, such as sausages, meat pies, beefburgers, etc., contain considerable amounts of fat in the ingredients, which increase the energy content of these items. There is pressure on the food manufacturers to use less fat in these foods; lower-fat sausages and beefburgers are now available in Britain, and other new products of this type are likely to appear on the market. This is in line with a growing awareness of the damaging effects of a high fat intake.

Protein

Most people think of meat as primarily a supplier of protein. This is emphasized in Fig. 10.2: meat provides more protein in the British diet (31%) than any other food group in the Survey. This perhaps reflects the British view of a traditional meal as containing 'meat and two veg'. This is still strongly upheld in many, more traditional, households. There is, however, a growing section of the British population that eats meat less often, and some households have become completely vegetarian, eating no meat at all. This is reflected in the National Food Survey, which shows a progressive fall in meat consumption in Britain.

Many communities around the world eat little or no meat already, although there are also those which eat more than we do in Britain. One of the major influences on meat consumption is cost; in most societies less meat is eaten as income declines. It would be better for health if meat intake was reduced and seen as an added extra to the meal, rather than its central feature. The diet could then contain less fat and perhaps more dietary fibre from the vegetables which might replace the meat.

Fat

The fat obtained from meat makes the second largest contribution to the total fat intake in Britain. Meat fat contains predominantly saturated fatty acids. The actual proportions of fat in meat differ between different animals, and also between cuts of meat. The most saturated meat fat comes from beef and lamb, followed by pork, then poultry and game (i.e. birds and animals not normally reared by farming techniques, but killed in their natural habitat). British butchering methods have traditionally cut meat so that quite a large amount of integral fat is included within the joints. European-style butchering removes more of this fat from meat such as beef, pork and lamb and achieves leaner cuts. Most of the fat in poultry lies under the skin and so is much easier to remove. Game, which lives a natural life in open spaces, has little body fat, so the meat is considerably leaner.

Iron

When considering sources of iron, two food groups predominate: cereals and meats. The latter supply 21% of the intake. The iron in meat derives from the oxygen-carrying pigments found in the muscles of animals and in the blood remaining in meat. In consequence this iron is relatively readily absorbed from meat, as it is in the organic form (see Chapter 7). Most meat provides iron, although liver is the richest source. Liver, however, does not contribute significantly to the total, as it is rarely eaten by the majority of the population.

B vitamins

The three B vitamins listed in Table 10.1 are all supplied by meat. In particular, meat is an excellent source of nicotinic acid (34%). This arises from two constituents of meat: preformed nicotinic acid and tryptophan. The latter is converted to nicotinic acid by the body. Pork is the major supplier of thiamine in this group; most other meats are relatively poor in thiamine. However, the large overall intake of meat makes the total supply of thiamine reasonably high (14%). Riboflavin, at 18% of total intake, is mainly supplied by liver and meat products; the latter may contain offal and also egg and milk in pastry. It should be remembered that these water-soluble B vitamins are likely to be lost to an extent in cooking, especially in the form of juices dripping from the meat. To conserve as much of the vitamins as possible, meat juices should be used in gravies and sauces, so that they are not wasted.

Vitamin A

Although the total provision of this vitamin by the meat group is 37%, it is almost completely supplied by liver, which is an extremely rich source of the preformed vitamin (retinol). Thus despite the fact that many people do not eat liver, it still contributes significantly to the overall intake of vitamin A. However, the meat group will supply almost no vitamin A to the diet of the proportion of the population who do not eat liver, and their total intake of the vitamin may well be lower.

Other nutrients

Meat supplies none of the other nutrients in important amounts. It contains negligible amounts of carbohydrate, vitamins C and D. A small amount of calcium might be obtained from bone, especially when minute fragments of bone are eaten as contaminants of meat. Bone fragments may also be included in meat products made up from meat offcuts by food manufacturers, such as pies, pastries and burgers.

Total fish

Fish is very similar to meat in its nutrient composition. Differences may be seen between the oily fish such as mackerel and herring, and the white fish such as cod and plaice, particularly in the proportions of fat, with the former group having a much higher fat content. Both groups contain less fat and more water than meat, so the remaining nutrients become diluted.

As the bones of small fish (such as tinned sardines or pilchards, or small fresh fish) may be consumed whole, the calcium intake from a diet of fish may be higher than that from a meat diet. In addition, oily fish contain vitamin D, which is not found generally in meat. In fact, oily fish are one of the few dietary sources of this vitamin, and are particularly recommended for people who have little exposure to sunlight for the normal synthesis of the vitamin in the skin (Fig. 10.3).

Recently oily fish have been gaining favour as a 'healthy' food, in relation to heart disease. This is linked to their high content of some very unsaturated long-chain fatty acids, which are thought to be of benefit in the circulation. However, despite these benefits, the consumption of fish is relatively low in the UK, and the fish eaten is increasingly pre-prepared fish, rather than the wet fish available from fishmongers.

In considering the nutrients available from fish of all types (Fig. 10.3), the only notable contribution by this group is to the vitamin D intake (14%). As with vitamin A in liver, this applies only to the minority of the population who regularly eat mackerel, herring, or tinned fatty fish, like sardines, pilchards and tuna. Although other nutrients are provided, their significance in the diet is minimal.

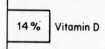

14 %   Vitamin D

Fig. 10.3   Nutrients provided by fish as a percentage of total diet (see Table 10.1).

Eggs

It is the egg of the chicken which is commonly eaten in Britain. An egg contains the majority of nutrients necessary for the development of a chick; thus eggs provide a wide range of nutrients. However, the overall contribution they make to the UK diet is small (Fig. 10.4). This reflects the decreasing importance of eggs, especially as part of the traditional cooked breakfast. Only vitamin D is noteworthy: eggs supply 12% of the dietary intake of this vitamin and, as with oily fish, their consumption is to be encouraged in the diet of people who may have little exposure to sunlight.

The inclusion of eggs in the diet has been discouraged by many 'healthy eating' reports, particularly those published in the USA. This is associated with their high

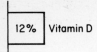

Fig. 10.4   Nutrients provided by eggs as a percentage of total diet (see Table 10.1).

cholesterol content which had been thought to elevate plasma cholesterol levels and so increase the risks of heart disease. Although it is probably wise for those with high blood cholesterol levels to keep to a maximum of 2 or 3 eggs per week, there is little evidence that a moderate intake of eggs (perhaps 5 to 6 per week) is in any way hazardous to the majority. Nevertheless, fears about high cholesterol intakes may have contributed to the present low egg consumption in the UK.

Fats

Included in this section are all the culinary fats used in the UK: butter, margarine, oils, lard and dripping. These fats serve different purposes – some are used to spread on bread and others are used principally in cooking. Only four nutrients are provided in significant amounts by the dietary fats: energy, fat and the fat-soluble vitamins, A and D (Fig. 10.5).

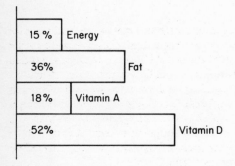

Fig. 10.5   Nutrients provided by fats as a percentage of total diet (see Table 10.1).

Energy

Culinary fats provide about 15% of the total intake of energy; it is important to remember, however, that energy from fat is also obtained in many other foods (as already mentioned in the sections on meat and dairy products). Fats are a very concentrated form of energy, supplying 37 kJ/g of pure fat. Most culinary fats (with the exception of low-fat spreads) are virtually water-free. This is unusual, as most other categories of food contain up to 80% water. Therefore, a small amount of fat can add a large amount of energy to the diet. Conversely, even a small reduction in the use of fat can cut the energy intake quite significantly.

Culinary fats can be modified without affecting many other nutrients. For example, the low-fat spreads on the market are simply a mixture of fats that have been diluted with water and then made into a stable, spreadable emulsion. In this way, it is possible to cut down on the energy from fat, without risking any of the other nutrients.

Fat

This group supplies 36% of the average UK intake of fat. This figure does not, however, differentiate between the saturated and unsaturated fatty acids in the diet. The Survey shows that the ratio of polyunsaturated fatty acids to saturated fatty acids (P:S ratio) is currently 0.3. This gives a measure of the relative proportions of these two types of fats in the diet.

As mentioned above, a reduction in the intake of fats could be reasonably easily achieved by using less fat on bread and in cooking, or by using a low-fat spread. The practical possibilities for reducing fat intakes are considered in Chapter 11.

Fats in food increase the palatability of the diet, so people who try to cut down may find that initially foods seem less acceptable. The effect of fat on palatability is perhaps best seen in the high appeal of fried foods. The traditional British meal of 'fish and chips' is high in fat, from the fat taken up during deep-frying. In parts of Scotland and Northern Ireland the 'frying' tradition is very strong and has even embraced such non-British foods as pizza, as well as the usual bread, black pudding and bacon. Not surprisingly, the total fat intake in these regions is high.

Vitamin A

The vitamin A in the fats group comes from butter and margarine, and supplies 18% of total intake. In butter it is found both as preformed retinol as well as some β-carotene, which is converted to retinol by the body. However, the levels found in butter vary seasonally depending on the content in milk, which in turn reflects the diet of the cow. A much more consistent and higher level of the vitamin is found in margarine (and low-fat spreads). This is because the vitamin is added as a legal requirement at a level of 800 to 1000 μg/100 g to all margarine sold at the retail level. Therefore it is possible to obtain a useful supply of vitamin A from margarine. It is worthwhile to note that catering packs of margarine are not covered by the regulations on the addition of vitamins A and D.

Vitamin D

The fats group is the single most important source of vitamin D in the diet. As with vitamin A, most of it comes from margarine, to which it is added as a legal requirement in the UK, at a level of 7 to 9 μg/100 g. For people who get little exposure to sunlight, and for all British people in the winter, margarines make an important contribution to the dietary vitamin D. The vitamin is fairly stable to heat, but if the margarine is heated to a very high temperature some vitamin D may be destroyed. People from the Indian subcontinent may use margarine to form their own type of cooking fat, called *ghee*. This will contain useful amounts of vitamin D if it is made with some margarine, rather than the traditional 100% butter.

Vitamin D in butter is seasonally variable, again reflecting the changing exposure of cows to sunlight, and the quality of their diet, which influences the content of the vitamin in milk, and subsequently in butter. Summer butters and milks tend to be richer in both of these fat-soluble vitamins.

Fats thus supply both the fat-soluble vitamins, A and D, in important amounts. Lack of fat in the diet can significantly reduce their absorption.

Sugars and preserves

It is frequently stated that the British have a 'sweet tooth', and consume a large amount of sugar. This is confirmed by the annual consumption figure for the UK for sugar, which is 38 kg per head (1980 figure). However, in the Survey, sugar eaten as such and in the form of preserves appears to supply only 8% of the energy and 18% of the total carbohydrate intake (Fig. 10.6). It is very important to emphasize here that only foods brought into the household are considered by the Survey, which therefore excludes many of the confectionery items which are bought and eaten outside the home. Also, a considerable amount of sugar is included in many manufactured foods, and therefore appears in some of the other NFS categories. It has been said that over the last 30 years total sugar consumption in the UK has remained fairly stable. However, the amount of sugar as such being bought and used at home has progressively declined. The reason for this apparent anomaly is that more and more sugar is being added to processed and manufactured foods, making the total intake fairly constant over the whole period.

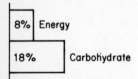

Fig. 10.6   Nutrients provided by sugars and preserves as a percentage of total diet (see Table 10.1).

Carbohydrate

Of the total carbohydrate, 18% is supplied by the sugars and preserves group. The carbohydrate consists predominantly of simple sugars, mainly sucrose, together with small amounts of fructose and glucose. This is the form of carbohydrate that most of the 'healthy eating' advice suggests should be reduced: this is discussed further in Chapter 11.

The sugars and preserves group adds little to the diet, apart from carbohydrates and their associated energy. Indeed, these foods are a very good example of high energy, low nutrient density foods. Another way of describing them would be as suppliers of 'empty energy' (the term 'empty energy' is explained more fully in Chapter 2).

Any other nutrients which might be present, such as vitamin C in jam, or B vitamins and minerals in honey, are there in such small amounts that for practical purposes they make a negligible contribution to the diet.

Vegetables

This is a very diverse group, containing potatoes, one of the major UK staple foods, as well as the pulse vegetables (peas and beans), roots, green leafy vegetables and salad vegetables. All have different nutrient contents, and are eaten in varying amounts. For example, potatoes may feature in the diet every day, or at least several times each week, whereas salad items may occur only in a few of the summer months. Conversely, other vegetables like parsnips or brussel sprouts are typical of the winter, and their appearance in the summer would be unusual. In total, the vegetables provide energy, protein, carbohydrate, iron, B vitamins, vitamin C and vitamin A (Fig. 10.7). When considering the nutrient content of vegetables, however, it must be remembered that their main constituent is water. This even applies to vegetables which are bought dried, but have to be rehydrated before eating.

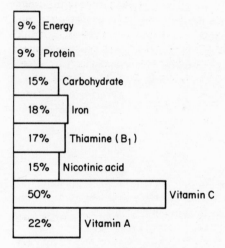

9%	Energy
9%	Protein
15%	Carbohydrate
18%	Iron
17%	Thiamine (B$_1$)
15%	Nicotinic acid
50%	Vitamin C
22%	Vitamin A

Fig. 10.7   Nutrients provided by vegetables as a percentage of total diet (see Table 10.1).

Energy

Only 9% of total energy comes from this group. Perhaps it is surprising that a group which includes potatoes, one of our staple foods in Britain, actually supplies such a relatively small amount of energy. Indeed, it emphasizes the fact that the potato has been much maligned as a high-energy, fattening food! This depends very much on whether the potato is roasted or deep-fried in fat, cooked with butter or mashed with milk and butter. Plain, boiled or baked potatoes are certainly not high in energy and make little impact on total energy intakes, even if eaten daily!

Protein

Most vegetables supply little protein. The overall figure of 9% of protein is derived partly from protein in potatoes and also from vegetable products. This includes canned baked beans and other canned vegetables such as peas. The potato itself is not rich in protein, but the amount eaten ensures that it does make a contribution. Peas, beans and other pulses are an important source of protein in vegetarian diets, where they can help to meet a significant proportion of the total protein needed. In many countries a large variety of these pulse vegetables is grown, dried and stored for use throughout the year; they act as the mainstay of the diet, along with a starchy root or cereal. Even in a meat-eater's diet, the inclusion of pulses will add to the protein intake. Pulses may also be sprouted; the product is high in vitamin C, further enhancing their nutritional value.

Carbohydrate

Vegetables contribute 15% to the total carbohydrate of the diet, most of this in the form of complex carbohydrates such as starch. Small amounts of the simple carbohydrates do occur in vegetables such as peas, onions and tomatoes, but this forms only a small proportion of the total. In recent years, it has been recognized that these complex carbohydrates in vegetables are an important item in a healthy diet. As a result, most 'healthy eating' advice promotes vegetables, because they are a low-energy source of carbohydrates, including those supplying dietary fibre. In addition, vegetables can be relatively inexpensive; by increasing the volume of a meal and thereby contributing to the satiety, vegetables can replace at least some of the more costly meat components. Further, the variety of vegetables and their colourful appearance can make this type of meal look very appetizing and attractive.

Iron

Iron is supplied in small amounts by most of the vegetables; it is mainly obtained from potatoes (due to the amount eaten) and vegetable products (for example baked beans). The iron in vegetables is in the inorganic form and as such is more difficult to absorb than the organic (animal foods) form. Further, salts such as iron oxalates may be formed in certain vegetables (spinach is particularly rich in oxalates), making the iron unavailable for absorption. On the positive side, however, many of the vegetables are rich in vitamin C, which promotes iron absorption. It is therefore important, especially in a vegetarian diet, that vegetables are not overcooked, thus preserving as much vitamin C as possible. This will facilitate the absorption of the vegetable-derived iron.

B vitamins

Vegetables supply all three of the B vitamins listed in the Survey, with nicotinic acid (15%) and thiamine (17%) being the more important. Potatoes and pulses (particularly the canned ones) are the major suppliers of these three vitamins; in addition, riboflavin is supplied by the green leafy vegetables, in small amounts.

All of these B vitamins are water-soluble and so are readily leached away by cooking. In addition, thiamine is heat-sensitive. A further problem arises when sodium bicarbonate is added to the cooking water to enhance the green colour of the leafy vegetables. This produces an alkaline environment, which further destroys the thiamine.

Generally, it is important that vegetables are not overcooked. Wherever possible, the cooking water should be used in another part of the meal, for instance in making gravy or as the basis of a soup. Vegetables that are not overcooked will also retain many of the other vitamins not considered in the Survey, such as folic acid and pyridoxine.

Vitamin C

Vegetables provide 50% of the total intake of this vitamin in the British household diet. By far the most important single source of vitamin C in this group is potatoes, providing 22% of the vitamin. This figure is an overall annual value. Potatoes contain more vitamin C when they are new and freshly harvested; the content declines on storage. Thus potatoes in the spring are relatively low in the vitamin. However, the large amount of potatoes eaten offsets their variable and sometimes low vitamin C content, so that they provide an important source of the vitamin. Other suppliers of vitamin C among the vegetables are the vegetable products, including canned vegetables, green leafy vegetables and tomatoes. Vitamin C is particularly vulnerable to loss if vegetables are overcooked or subsequently kept hot. Eating raw or lightly cooked vegetables is to be recommended in this context.

Where income is limited, potatoes may be the only source of vitamin C, rarely supplemented by another vegetable. A diet relying on the potato for vitamin C may be quite adequate most of the time. It does, however, run the risk of an insufficient intake of the vitamin, if the potatoes are badly cooked or kept hot for long periods of time. The potato may also be an inadequate source of vitamin C in the late winter or early spring, when the tubers have been stored for several months and their vitamin C content has declined. Instant potato powder is now generally enriched with vitamin C, since the manufacturing process reduces the existing levels; this type of potato may give a more reliable supply of the vitamin.

Vitamin A

No preformed retinol is provided by vegetables, but carotene contributes 22% of the total vitamin A intake. The single most important contributing vegetable here is the carrot, providing 14% of the vitamin A. It is an indication of the extremely high carotene levels in carrots that their contribution is so great. Although other vegetables such as tomatoes and green leafy vegetables also supply carotene, their actual significance in the total vitamin A intake, in general, is small.

Fruits

The fruit section includes citrus fruits, apples, pears, bananas, soft fruit and fruit products. However, despite their sweetness and apparent carbohydrate content, fruits add little to the overall carbohydrate in the diet. Their sole important contribution is to the total vitamin C (Fig. 10.8).

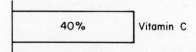

Fig. 10.8   Nutrients provided by fruits as a percentage of total diet (see Table 10.1).

Vitamin C

Of the total vitamin C, 40% is supplied by fruit, making it almost equal with vegetables in the provision of this vitamin. Citrus fruits provide almost 10% of this, a reflection of their richness in vitamin C rather than their frequency in the diet. A further 20% comes from 'other fruit and fruit products', which includes fruit juices rich in vitamin C. The most commonly eaten fruits – apples, pears and bananas – do not make a great contribution, as they are relatively poor in the vitamin.

An advantage of fruits over vegetables as a source of vitamin C is that they are generally eaten uncooked. This ensures better conservation of the vitamin, with no cooking losses. If fruit is cooked, the acidity protects the vitamin C, so there is little destruction of the vitamin.

Cereals

The cereal group of foods contains white and other breads, as well as flour and flour products (cakes, biscuits, pastries). In addition other cereals and cereal products such as breakfast cereals are considered. This is a major group, as it contains wheat and its products, which are the main UK staples. It is not surprising that a large percentage of the nutrient intake is supplied by this group. Significant nutrients are energy, protein, carbohydrate, calcium and iron, together with all the B vitamins included in the Survey (Fig. 10.9).

Notable nutrients missing from this group are fats and fat-soluble vitamins A and D. Any fat supplied by this group originates from the flour products, such as cakes, pastries, etc., which include fats in their manufacture. A small amount of vitamin D is also provided by the fortification of breakfast cereals, on a voluntary basis by some food manufacturers. In addition, no vitamin C is provided by the cereals group.

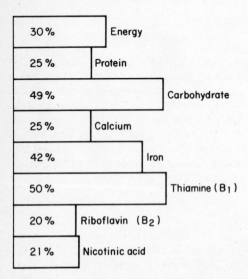

Fig. 10.9 Nutrients provided by cereals as a percentage of total diet (see Table 10.1).

Energy

Cereals provide 30% of the total energy intake in the UK. Over 13% of this comes from bread of all types, emphasizing its staple role in the British diet. Breakfast cereals also supply a consistent amount of energy; most people who eat these have them daily. Their popularity has increased in recent years, and they have far outstripped the 'bacon and egg' breakfast. The energy from cereals is mostly supplied by carbohydrates. Healthy eating advice promotes more cereal consumption, preferably in its less refined form. The common misconception that this cereal energy is particularly fattening is unfounded. However, if the cereal foods are eaten with large amounts of fat, sugar or cream, additional energy will be taken, which may lead to overweight. Plain bread, be it white, brown or wholemeal, is not high in energy.

Protein

Cereals are often disregarded as a source of protein, being seen as generally inferior to the animal products like meat and dairy produce. This is a mistaken view, since 25% of total protein comes from this group, putting it in second place amongst the sources of protein. It is true that the amino acid pattern of wheat is less like that of human tissues than, say, that of meat or milk. However, if the wheat is eaten with a small amount of another protein source – whether it is of plant or animal origin – then its quality is enhanced. This has been explained more fully in Chapter 6.

Many authorities agree that the diet should provide some 10 to 20% of its total energy as protein. This ensures that, on the one hand, enough protein is supplied for body needs, and on the other hand that excessive amounts are not eaten and wasted. Comparison of the cereals group with this ideal indicates that they supply 11% of energy as protein. This would suggest the cereals eaten are a very well-balanced item in our diet.

Carbohydrate

The majority of the energy supplied by cereals is in the form of carbohydrate. The group as a whole supplies 49% of all the carbohydrate in household diets, and is the single most important source of this nutrient. The survey does not subdivide the carbohydrate into simple and complex forms; thus it is not possible to comment on the dietary fibre content of the British diet in any detail. However, the majority of the carbohydrate supplied by cereals is in the complex form such as starch. Even in refined cereals, little carbohydrate will have been changed into simple forms such as monosaccharides and disaccharides. Therefore, cereal carbohydrate is in general to be recommended for a healthy diet.

Calcium

Slightly over 25% of calcium intake is obtained from the cereals group. In the unrefined form, wheat does contain a reasonable amount of calcium (38 mg per 100 g wholemeal flour), although its availability is probably reduced by the presence of dietary fibre and phytates. Refined wheat flour (less than 85%

extraction) has calcium added to it by law (at 235 to 390 mg per 100 g flour). As a result, products derived from this flour have a consistent calcium content. There has been considerable scientific debate about the need for this addition of calcium (and of iron, thiamine and nicotinic acid) to refined flour, at a time when the British diet is apparently nutritionally adequate. The most recent report of the Committee on Bread and Flour Regulations (1984) recommended that the additions should no longer be made. However, there followed pressure from organizations representing the poor and other groups. This is because people on a low food budget obtain more than the national average amounts of the four added nutrients from bread and flour products. If the additions were withdrawn, it would be these groups that would suffer disproportionately. Mainly for this reason, the nutritional additions will continue to be made for the foreseeable future at least.

Iron

The iron in cereals supplies almost 42% of the average intake of the mineral. A proportion of this is provided by the iron added, by law, to flour of less than 85% extraction (1.65 mg per 100 g of flour). Once again, those with the lowest incomes are more dependent on this iron than the average. It is for this reason that the addition of iron (like calcium) is to be continued. Iron is also added at the manufacturer's discretion to some breakfast cereals. Nevertheless, there is some doubt about the availability to the body of the iron added to flour. Studies performed on the absorption of this iron have shown that less than 2% may actually be available to the body cells.

As described in Chapter 7, iron absorption is affected by many other dietary components. Thus the iron from bread eaten with egg or tea may be hardly absorbed at all. On the other hand, the iron in a flour product such as pastry, eaten with vegetables and maybe accompanied by wine, or in toast eaten for breakfast and preceded by orange juice (both orange juice and vegetables supplying vitamin C), will have its absorption enhanced. Taking all of these aspects into account, the cereals group remains the most important source of iron. Whether it is utilized by the body as efficiently as the iron from meat is unlikely. On the other hand, if it forms the major source of iron in the diet, either of vegetarians or of those on a limited budget who eat little meat, every effort should be made to enhance its absorption rate.

B vitamins

All three of the B vitamins reported in the Survey are supplied in important amounts by the cereals group. Thiamine, of which 50% comes from cereal foods, is the most important. Thiamine occurs naturally in wheat and other cereals, predominantly in the outer layers of the grain. Consequently it is lost disproportionately during milling and refining of cereals, as in the production of white flour from wheat. However, further thiamine is obtained by addition at the mill, as required by law (0.24 mg per 100 g flour). This added thiamine is especially valuable for those on a low income. Many breakfast cereals are fortified with thiamine, which contributes an important amount to the thiamine intake of people who eat them regularly, especially children.

Breakfast cereals manufactured from whole grains, such as wholewheat cereals and those made from whole rice, oats or maize, contain most of the naturally occurring nutrients already. Any added nutrients included by the manufacturer therefore enhance the pre-existing nutritional value.

It is fortunate that cereals, which are an important source of carbohydrate, also supply thiamine in large amounts, as the vitamin is closely associated with carbohydrate metabolism. An increased intake of carbohydrate increases the need for thiamine. Thus cereals are 'balanced' in terms of their carbohydrate and thiamine ratio, as they are for their protein and energy ratio.

Riboflavin and nicotinic acid (20% and 21% of the total supply, respectively) are supplied largely by the cereal products in this group. This originates from the fortification of breakfast cereals, as well as the use of other foods containing these vitamins (such as eggs and milk) in the making of cereal products. Cereals themselves are not an especially rich source of either of these two vitamins.

Nevertheless, when considered as a complete group, cereals and their products make an important contribution to the dietary intake of all three of the B vitamins studied here.

Beverages

This group includes tea, coffee, cocoa and carbonated drinks, but excludes fruit juices and milk, which are considered in the fruit and dairy produce sections respectively. The National Food Survey does not consider alcoholic beverages, as these are more often bought and consumed outside the household, and therefore do not enter into the sphere of items considered in detail by the Survey. However, the amount of energy provided by alcoholic beverages is considered; in 1984 this amounted to 630 kJ per head per day. Alcoholic beverages provide no other significant nutrients.

Very little nutritional value is supplied by the non-alcoholic beverages. This is because they are composed largely of water, or of milk, in the case of 'bedtime' drinks such as cocoa. These beverages can provide a small amount of riboflavin and nicotinic acid. For people who drink large amounts of tea, coffee or cocoa, these may actually make an important addition to the day's intake. However, their vitamin content should be viewed in perspective. In comparison with other foods, they provide very small amounts of nutrients. They should be viewed therefore as pleasant additions to the diet, rather than as major contributors of nutrients. For example, it would not be possible for these beverages to meet the daily needs for either riboflavin or nicotinic acid of an individual.

Conclusion

The current typical British diet has been described in this chapter. The discussion has not taken into account individual household variation, nor the distribution of foods within households. The framework of the National Food Survey has been used to describe the major nutritional features of food groups in the diet and to highlight the importance of particular nutrients within these groups. As the sampling technique used by the Survey aims to make it representative of the population of households in the UK, so its results indicate the typical, average household consumption. For further information on the data presented here, the reader is referred to the National Food Survey Committee reports, published annually.

Although the nutritional value of the diet has been discussed in relation to statistics referring to the United Kingdom, the same food groups appear in most other national diets. It follows that the nutrients they supply will also be the same. Differences occur only in the proportions of the different foods eaten, and hence the relative importance of the differing food groups in supplying particular nutrients. The actual nutrients supplied remain the same.

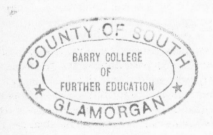

11

The British Diet – What Could It Provide?

A comparison of the foods found in the present-day British diet, and the levels of nutrients recommended for the British population, shows that on the whole these intakes are satisfactory.

However, if the incidence of various diseases in the western world is considered, it seems that perhaps the diet is not altogether satisfactory. There is a widespread belief among nutritionists, epidemiologists and doctors that many diseases are diet-related, and that a change in the diet would reduce their incidence. The diseases involved include cardiovascular diseases (resulting in angina, heart attacks and strokes); intestinal disorders (such as cancer of the colon, gallstones, constipation and diverticular disease); obesity and dental caries. Many of these result in death, or at best disability, so it is desirable to try to prevent or reduce this 'avoidable' disease.

The aim of the NACNE report in 1983 was to present guidelines for the British diet that would result in better health and thereby reduce the incidence of the diseases listed above.

Background to the NACNE report

The committee that produced this report included representatives from practising nutritionists, the food industry, government departments, health educators and academics. It was therefore broadly representative of nutritional interest groups. The committee produced a consensus view after considering the findings of a number of reports published by specialist bodies in the previous ten years. On this basis, they recommended more specific changes to the British diet than had ever been suggested in the past. This reflected a feeling that the population actually wanted more specific targets for food intakes, rather than general comments about 'less of this' or 'more of that'.

Two sets of recommendations were made: for the 1980s (short term) and up to the year 2000 (long term). This approach recognizes the radical changes which have to occur in the eating patterns of some of the population. By allowing a 15-year interval for the full changes to be incorporated into the eating patterns, the guidelines allow time for the educators to put across the new thinking on food and nutrition. It also allows time for food manufacturers to respond to an altered demand, by producing new, healthier foods. A third change which may take place over the next 15 years is in some government policies. For example, changes on the laws of food labelling are already being made: these will provide clearer inform-ation to the public, and serve as part of the process of education.

What are the NACNE recommendations?

The figures in Table 11.1 are meant as average intakes and therefore do not necessarily imply that everyone should conform to these. Neither are they maximum or minimum levels.

Table 11.1 Short-term and long-term nutritional guidelines, as proposed by the NACNE Report (1983).

Dietary component	Short-term recommendation	Long-term recommendation
Energy		Energy intake should be sufficient to maintain optimal body weight, with exercise.
Total fat	To be reduced to 34% of total energy intake.	To be reduced to 30% of total energy intake.
Saturated fat	To fall to 15% of total energy intake.	To fall to 10% of total energy intake.
Polyunsaturated fat	To increase slightly, to 5% of total energy, to offset some of the fall in saturated fat sources. P:S ratio to rise to 0.32.	No specific recommendation made; polyunsaturated fat intake will automatically form a greater proportion of the total if the other recommendations are met.
Sucrose	To fall to 34 kg per head per year.	To fall to 20 kg per head per year; of this no more than 10 kg should be from snacks.
Dietary fibre	To increase to 25 g per head per day.	To increase to 30 g per head per day.
Salt	To be reduced by 1 g per day.	To reduce by 3 g per day.
Alcohol	Intakes should move towards a level of no more than 5% of total energy.	Levels should not exceed 4% of total energy.
Protein		Intakes should be maintained, but a greater proportion should come from vegetable protein sources.

Energy

The committee recommended that total energy intakes should be matched to energy output. Whilst recognizing that overweight is a problem, it was not recommended that overall food intakes be reduced. An alteration of the balance between carbohydrate and fat in the diet is suggested as an alternative; with higher carbohydrate intake and less fat, this results in a fall in total energy intake, since fat contains more energy per gram than carbohydrate. The committee very strongly recommended that the notion of carbohydrates as being 'fattening' should be discouraged.

Further, considerable encouragement was given to the taking of exercise as a means of increasing the energy output to match the higher energy intake. This was thought to be desirable at all ages, not just for children and young adults, but throughout the age span, and even for the elderly. If the exercise habit starts young, it will persist throughout life.

Fats

(1) *Total fat.* Most authorities agree that the high total fat intakes in western countries, including Britain, are in part responsible for the incidence of vascular diseases, resulting in heart disease and strokes. The average plasma cholesterol level in a population group is a reflection of the proportion of fat in their diet. To reduce the plasma cholesterol to a level that is associated with a relatively low risk of heart disease (less than 230 mg/dl) requires that total fat intake should be in the region of 30% of total energy. This level of intake is recommended as being acceptable within the British dietary pattern.

(2) *Saturated fats and polyunsaturated fatty acids (PUFA).* There has been considerable controversy over the relative dangers and merits of saturated fatty acids and PUFA, with the result that many people are very confused. The NACNE report suggests that it is the saturated fat component of the diet that should be cut, to 10% of total energy, since this is the level recommended by other bodies concerned with the prevention of heart disease. Unfortunately such a reduction would significantly affect the palatability of the diet (see Chapter 5). It is therefore recognized that some of the saturated fats (especially butter and other culinary fats) may be replaced by more polyunsaturated products (some soft magarines and oils). However, no recommendation is made specifically to increase PUFA intakes, as there is still doubt about the safety, desirability and feasibility of such a measure.

(3) *Cholesterol.* No recommendations are made for reductions in dietary cholesterol. There is little evidence that dietary cholesterol as such has any major health implications. A reduction in total and saturated fat is much more effective and important for health. It will also have the effect of automatically reducing cholesterol intakes, as this nutrient is found in foods containing saturated fats.

Carbohydrates

(1) *Refined carbohydrates.* Sucrose is the major refined carbohydrate in the western diet. It is eaten both in the form of 'visible' added sugar and 'invisible' sugar, incorporated into many prepared foods such as cakes and biscuits. It is also included in many manufactured foods as a preservative or flavour enhancer; it thus finds its way into many foods that one might not expect to contain sugar. Sugar contributes energy to the diet without adding other nutrients; it is therefore a source of 'empty energy' and as such may contribute to overweight. In addition, sugar eaten at frequent intervals throughout the day promotes dental caries, which is prevalent in the West (see Chapter 16), and is increasing in many developing countries, as the taste for western refined products spreads to the towns and cities of the Third World.

The NACNE report recommends a reduction of sugar intake to a total of 20 kg per head per year. The suggested proportion is that half of this sugar may be present in main meals, and the remainder eaten as snacks.

(2) *Unrefined carbohydrates.* Epidemiological evidence on intakes of dietary fibre and disease incidence from various countries, together with studies in

vegetarians, points to a reduced incidence of bowel disorders and – in the latter group – benefits in relation to heart disease and body weight, linked to a higher intake of dietary fibre (see Chapter 17). On the basis of such data, the committee recommended an increase in dietary fibre intake to 30 g per day. This additional fibre should be taken in the form of whole (as opposed to refined) foods, such as vegetables, fruit and whole-grain cereals and their products. Bran, a 'refined' form of dietary fibre, is not recommended, as this does not contain any additional minerals or vitamins to compensate for a reduced absorption of some of these nutrients, which can occur with a higher intake level of dietary fibre.

Salt

Epidemiological findings show a positive correlation between salt intake and average blood pressure in a population. The NACNE report recommends a reduction in the salt intake to 9 g per day, from the current estimated level of 12 g per day. This is designed to reduce the average blood pressure of the whole population, and thereby cause a reduction in the number of people with high blood pressure. As high blood pressure considerably increases the risk of strokes and heart disease, a fall in the number of these diseases is envisaged. The report points out that such a reduction in salt intakes will require some action by the food manufacturers. This is because 75% of the current salt intake is estimated to come from processed and manufactured foods. Addition of salt in cooking and at the table provides only a small proportion of the total intake.

Alcohol

The committee did not consider the question of alcohol intake in detail; however the recommendations of other organizations are presented. It is recommended that average alcohol intake should not exceed 4% of the total energy. This would be equivalent to slightly less than 20 g alcohol per day, or less than 1 pint of beer, 2 measures of spirits or 2 glasses of wine. The maximum regular intake should not exceed 80 g alcohol per day (or 4 pints of beer per day).

Summary

In summary the NACNE report recommended that in Britain we should eat:
    less fat (especially saturated fat)
    less sugar
    more unrefined, whole carbohydrate
    less alcohol
    less salt.

What does this mean in practical terms?

Chapter 10 described which food groups are the main providers of particular nutrients in the existing UK diet. By looking at the current pattern of intake, areas can be pinpointed in which amounts of particular foods need to be cut down, and others increased. In this way a healthier diet can be achieved, using familiar foods, but selecting them in different proportions. For each of the nutrients considered by NACNE, ways to achieve the targets by modification of the existing food intake are described below.

Reduce fat

The NACNE recommendations are to reduce total fat, reduce saturated fats and increase total polyunsaturated fats.

From Table 10.1 on p. 100 it can be seen that the foods which currently provide most fat are (in decreasing order of importance): culinary fats, meat and the dairy produce group. Together these groups provide 80% of all the fat eaten in the UK. The meat and dairy produce groups are the main suppliers of saturated fats, although some of these also come from the culinary fats group. It should, however, be remembered that the culinary fats group – if carefully selected – can supply important amounts of polyunsaturated fats.

An overall reduction in the intake of all three of the above-mentioned groups is desirable. Some practical hints might be:

(1) Use less fat in cooking: grill or bake foods rather than frying or deep frying. If fat is used in cooking, try to use unsaturated oils and margarines, rather than lard or butter. Choose the pure vegetable oils (such as soya, corn or sunflower oils) as they contain most polyunsaturated fats. The blended and mixed oils ('vegetable oil'), as well as groundnut oil, have rather more saturated fat in them. Similarly, margarines contain some saturated (hardened) fats, which have been introduced to convert them from an oil into a solid substance in the manufacturing process. Choose those which are labelled 'high in polyunsaturates', as they contain more than 45% of total fat as polyunsaturates and 25% or less of the fat will be saturated.

(2) Spread less fat on bread; this can mean using a scraping of a fat such as butter or margarine, or perhaps changing to one of the low-fat spreads. Some bread, if it accompanies other foods, can be eaten with no fat on it at all.

(3) Eat fewer made-up, processed products, which contain a lot of fat; some biscuits, cakes and pastries have a large amount of 'hidden' fat.

(4) Eat less meat: even apparently lean meat has quite a high fat content. Choose the leanest cuts, trimmed of surrounding fat, including lean gammon, stews and liver. Some may be more expensive, but if you are eating less meat, the overall costs need not be higher. It is also better to choose those varieties of meat that have a lower saturated fat content, such as chicken, other poultry and game. The fat in pork is also less saturated than that in beef or lamb.

A healthier alternative to meat is fish in all forms. The fats they contain are poly-unsaturated and the total fat content is less. Replacing some of the meat with fish dishes, is a recommended, healthier alternative.

Meat dishes containing smaller amounts of meat can be made more substantial by the addition of extra vegetables, to make dishes such as shepherd's pie (meat and potatoes) stews with vegetables or spaghetti dishes. Traditional Indian and Chinese cuisines use meat very sparingly and add many different vegetables to en-hance their meat dishes.

(5) Eat fewer prepared meat dishes, such as pasties, pies, sausages and tinned meats like luncheon meat; they are usually high in fat (often saturated). Fat incor-porated into a dish in this way cannot be removed easily, nor can it be seen; the consumer therefore has almost no control over fat intake from these foods. In

addition, any pastry forming part of the dish may be high in fat (e.g. flaky pastry used as a pie shell).

(6) Switch to the least fatty types of milk, cream and cheese that are acceptable. Semi-skimmed milk has half of the total milk fat removed, but tastes very similar to whole milk. Skimmed milk is even lower in fat, and makes little difference to the taste of foods when used in cooking. Some find it tastes rather 'thin' for use as a drink or in tea and coffee. However, it can easily become accepted as part of the diet. Full-fat milk then becomes excessively rich to the palate!

Single cream has less fat than whipping or double cream and can often be used in their place. However, other low-fat alternatives such as natural yoghurt may be used successfully.

Lower-fat cheeses, such as cottage cheese, are a suitable alternative for some uses. In addition 'half-fat' hard cheeses of the Cheddar variety are also available, where a firm cheese is needed. Some of these have an acceptable taste and texture; others are rather dry and do not adequately at present resemble their full-fat counterparts. They are, however, very useful in cooking, where a lower-fat cheese can significantly reduce the fat content of a dish.

(7) Polyunsaturated fats are found in vegetables in small amounts (especially in the growing tips, e.g. broccoli), in whole cereal grains (and their products) and in nuts. All of these foods are therefore recommended to be eaten in increased amounts, to produce an increase in the polyunsaturated fat intake. This can serve to offset some of the energy loss resulting from a reduction in the other fat-rich foods.

All of these changes, which aim to reduce the dietary intake of total and saturated fats, also result in a decrease in the cholesterol content of the diet. This will always be the case, except where egg intake is increased to compensate for a reduced meat content in the diet.

Reduce sugar

In Britain, we eat almost 1 kg of sugar per head per week. Only a third of this is actually brought into the household as packet sugar; the remainder is eaten in processed foods and sweets or confectionery. Sweet consumption averages 200 g per person per week.

While the amount of 'packet' sugar consumed has been steadily falling, that eaten in processed and manufactured foods has increased. Sugar is now added to a large array of packeted and tinned foods, in one guise or another. Label-readers will find sugar, sucrose, glucose, fructose, maltose, syrup, invert sugar as just some of the possible variants on the same theme. Brown sugar is frequently only coloured white sugar, and therefore possesses no nutritional advantage. 'Raw cane sugar' does contain some additional nutrients, present in the original sugar cane, but the quantities are too small to be of any significance.

All sugar provides energy, which can be rapidly available to the body due to the simplicity of sugar digestion. However, this energy, separated from any other nutrients, is just 'empty energy' and serves either to supply unnecessary surplus energy, or dilutes the rest of the diet, putting other nutrients at risk. In addition, sugar contributes to tooth decay, and may also be in part responsible for the development of diabetes mellitus in later life.

It would be almost impossible to cut out sugar completely from the normal western diet. Most nutritionists do not believe that such a drastic measure is actually necessary. Some practical hints to reduce sugar intake include:

(1) Cut out the use of sugar in beverages such as tea and coffee; best of all get used to their natural tastes, but if necessary, use an artificial sweetener. 'Low calorie' soft drinks, taken in moderation, are also better than the sugar-laden normal squashes and colas. Natural fruit juices, such as orange, grapefruit, apple and pineapple are even better.

(2) Limit the intake of sweets and confectionery. They do not have to be eliminated altogether, but perhaps seen as a special, occasional treat, rather than as a daily necessity of life. For children in particular it is best to avoid this habit of eating sweets. Parental example, and a positive attitude that the child is in no way being deprived, are a help. (What the child may be deprived of is bad teeth and ill-health in later life!) It is also better for dental health if sweets are eaten as part of a meal, and on perhaps just one day each week, rather than at more frequent intervals.

(3) Change to healthier snack foods. Avoid sugar-rich biscuits, sweets and confectionery: choose fresh and dried fruit, nuts or low-fat crisps instead.

(4) Look at the labels of tinned or packeted foods. If sugar (in any of its disguises) occurs as one of the first few listed ingredients – avoid that food!

(5) Use the sweetness of fruit to flavour sweet dishes, such as puddings: they will need less sugar in the recipe and will be healthier.

Increase unrefined carbohydrate

The changes discussed so far, cutting down on fat and sugar, may well result in a fall in total energy intake. The NACNE report does not see this as a desirable goal, and recommends that energy intakes be maintained. This additional energy must be obtained from other foods. Unrefined, complex carbohydrate sources are suggested to fill this gap. These are the foods commonly described as 'starchy' foods. Although Table 10.1 does not differentiate between simple and complex carbohydrates, it is known that the majority of the latter comes from cereals (48%) and some from vegetables (15%). It is these two groups that should be used to compensate for the energy reduction following a fall in fat and sugar intakes.

For decades, carbohydrates have had the reputation of being 'fattening', and therefore to be avoided. This view of 'wicked carbohydrates' persists still, despite the recognition recently that it is only some carbohydrates, namely the refined sugars, that are a source of empty energy and so of doubtful nutritional value. Quite rational people still believe that large amounts of weight will be gained by eating even small amounts of bread and potatoes. This belief is unfounded, but nevertheless deeply held; it can present a major obstacle to increasing intakes of cereals and vegetables. So what should the advice be?

(1) More bread. Ideally, more wholemeal bread ought to be included in the diet: six slices or more per day. Many varieties of bread are sold in the UK, with a confusing array of names. These include wholemeal (wholewheat), brown, wheatmeal, granary, wheatgerm, high-fibre bread and white bread. Apart from the first, none of these varieties contain all the nutrients of the wheat grain and therefore they are nutritionally less good. However, they still make a useful contribution to

the diet; and even white bread, which contains 72% of the original cereal, should be eaten in increased amounts by those people who are not willing to eat wholemeal bread. In fact, any bread is better than no bread. Of course, a point to beware is putting large quantities of fat and/or sweet things on the bread. A good quality, fresh loaf of bread requires little embellishment.

(2) More cereals and cereal products. These items should be increased in the diet. This includes eating more pasta or noodles, made up into a variety of dishes, as well as rice. Obviously, it is better to eat these in their wholegrain form (wholemeal pasta, brown rice), but these tend to be less widely available and more expensive. As with bread, more pasta and rice of whatever type is better than none.

Pastas and rice are an interesting alternative around which to base a meal. They can be made more varied with a large variety of sauces, based on small amounts of meat with vegetables, or with cheese and eggs. Many famous national cuisines include pasta, notably the Chinese and Italian. Both of these countries have much lower incidence of the 'Western diseases' than we do in Britain.

(3) More vegetables, all types. Potatoes are one of our major staple foods in the UK. However, the amounts eaten are much less than in the past. Many people eat potatoes most frequently in the form of chips, fried in fat. The vitamin C content of potatoes is preserved better by this means of cooking than by boiling and subsequent mashing. However chips contain a significant amount of fat, absorbed during the cooking. This contributes to their flavour and palatability, but also to their energy content! The newer 'oven chips' have a lower fat content, so in these terms are 'healthier'. By far the healthiest way of eating potatoes is to cook and eat them in their skins. More 'jacket potatoes' are being eaten in the West, as a result of increasing ownership of microwave ovens. In these, jacket potatoes are quick and economical to prepare and therefore occur as a more frequent menu item. They have also been successfully introduced into school meals, as a competing attraction against the ubiquitous chip.

In general, the range of vegetables eaten by the British population is narrow. This is a pity, since there are very many different vegetables available, and these could be used to add considerable variety to meals. They are usually colourful, with interesting shapes and textures, and should never be monotonous. Unfortunately, it is very easy to get into the habit of eating only the same three or four vegetables over and over again. No wonder they become boring!

As well as using more of the fresh vegetables commonly grown in this country, more use could be made of the dried pulse vegetables: peas, beans and lentils. There seems to be much ignorance about how to use these dried pulses. Rules about soaking and boiling tend to be off-putting, so that these nutritionally valuable products are only rarely used. Even then, it may be once or twice a year as part of a soup on a cold winter's day, rather than as a vegetable in a main meal. Some manufacturers are now producing canned pulses, such as red kidney beans, chick peas, etc. These are certainly useful as an introduction, but can be much more expensive than using the dried products. They do have the advantage of being considerably more convenient.

Whatever vegetables are eaten, it is important that they are not overcooked, so their nutrients are preserved, and the vegetables keep their integrity and shape.

As with bread and other foods that have been described, more of any vegetable is to be recommended.

Less alcohol

The National Food Survey does not include alcohol in its results, so that total energy figures in all of its tables are exclusive of alcoholic beverages.

The consumption of alcohol in Britain varies widely between individuals, and also between different parts of the country. Estimates suggest that the average intake ranges from 4 to 9% of average total energy. This reflects an increase in the consumption of alcohol over the last twenty years. A contributory factor in this has been the fall in the relative cost of many alcoholic beverages, in relation to other foods. Health professionals are in agreement over the adverse effects on health (and on other aspects of life) of excessive intakes of alcohol. Complete abstinence, however, is not recommended. Firstly, for many people it is not practical. Also it appears that mortality from certain diseases, especially of the cardiovascular system, is less in those who take a regular, moderate amount of alcohol.

In terms of actual numbers of drinks, the NACNE report suggests that the mean alcohol intake should be less than 1 pint of beer per day. The maximum regular intake should not be more than 4 pints of beer per day. Many people drink more than this, and it is this section of society whose health would improve if they were to cut their intake to less than 4 pints of beer (or its equivalent) per day. On the other hand, the moderate drinker appears to be in line with the NACNE proposals.

Less salt

Much of the salt we eat is contained in the manufactured foods in the diet. These include cheese, bacon, kippers and most canned and prepared foods. The original role of salt in many of these foods was that of a preservative. In many cases, this role has been taken over by newer preservative agents, but the addition of salt continues. In a typical British diet, containing a proportion of manufactured and convenience foods, about 75% of the salt originates from these foods, with the remaining 25% added in cooking or at the table.

On average about 20 times as much salt is eaten as is needed, and the basic biological need for salt could be met from the amounts of salt naturally occurring in foods such as meats or animal products in general. There is therefore no danger to health in reducing salt, even in warm weather. There is evidence of an advantage in terms of lowering of blood pressure in some individuals when they lower their salt intake.

How can salt intake be reduced in practice?

(1) Eat more unprocessed, fresh foods, especially vegetables: choose fresh meat and fish, rather than processed, packaged alternatives. Remember that common foods like cheese, bacon and some breakfast cereals are all high in salt.

(2) Read labels on packaged foods to see if they contain added salt. The earlier salt appears in a list of ingredients, the more there is in the food.

(3) Cut down on salt used in cooking. The taste buds will lose some of their 'addiction' to salt, so they no longer require it in large amounts. Use herbs and spices as alternative flavourings.

(4) Don't automatically add salt to food on the plate. Taste it first, to see if it needs salt. If you must add salt, use a salt shaker with a small hole. Use pepper as

an alternative seasoning. Many bottled sauces commonly used in Britain are high in salt (and sugar!). Children in particular should be discouraged from using them to prevent the salt habit developing.

The new healthy diet

There is no single correct way of achieving a diet along the guidelines laid down in the NACNE report. Individually, we can choose from a large selection of foods. The way this is done will depend on many factors, paticularly individual likes and dislikes. The NACNE recommendations do not state which specific foods should be eaten, or the amounts. Instead, they make suggestions about the proportions of items in the diet. As less of one food is eaten, so it can be replaced with more of something else. Table 11.2 gives a summary of some of the adjustments which could be made.

Table 11.2   Some practical examples of dietary adjustments that can be made to move towards the NACNE goals.

Meal	Eat more	Eat less

Breakfast	High-fibre breakfast cereals
	Wholemeal bread/toast
	Polyunsaturated margarines
	Low-fat spreads
	Skimmed or semiskimmed milk
	  with cereals/tea/coffee
	Low-sugar jam/marmalade
		Refined, sugary cereals
		White bread
		Butter and other margarines
		Whole milk/cream with cereals/
		  tea/coffee
		
		High-sugar preserves

Midmorning/ midafternoon	Fresh/dried fruit Fruit juice, low-calorie squash Tea/coffee with low-fat milk	Confectionery, biscuits Sugary drinks

Lunch	Wholemeal sandwiches with
	  low-fat fillings (lean meat,
	  low-fat cheese, salad)
	Fresh fruit
	Low-fat yoghurt
		Fried foods
		Pies/sausage rolls/pasties/chips
		Fatty cheeses, pâtés

Evening	Jacket potatoes/rice/pasta
	Lean meat/fish (grilled/baked)
	Vegetables (several)
	Fruit pie with wholemeal pastry
	  and yoghurt
		Mashed potatoes (with fat and
		  milk)
		Fatty meats/rich sauces
		Fried fish
		Buttered vegetables
		Rich puddings with cream
		High-fat cheese

Bedtime	Toast with low-fat spread Low-fat milk in drink	Biscuits Sugary drinks

Will the NACNE diet be expensive?

There is no reason why a healthier diet, approaching the nutritional proportions outlined by NACNE, should be more expensive than the present ordinary British diet. The total amounts of foods are similar; there is a trend to greater amounts of fruit, vegetables and cereals, which are usually cheaper than the meat and other fat-rich products, such as cheese, that they are intended to replace. On the other hand, wholemeal bread at present does cost more than white bread in Britain. Wholegrain rice and pastas are also more expensive. It requires changes in our eating habits, and therefore an increase in the demand for these foods, before their costs will fall. At the moment they are more expensive because fewer people are eating them, compared with their refined alternatives.

The diet may also be less convenient, because some of the pre-prepared foods are being discouraged. However, food manufacturers are becoming aware of this, and increasing numbers of healthier alternatives in a 'convenience' form are being marketed. On the other hand, some foods suggested by NACNE are more convenient: a jacket potato is very simple to cook; fresh fruit for pudding is much simpler than making a pie or some other cooked pudding. More bread is also suggested; putting together a sandwich is quicker and easier than making chips and frying eggs, bacon and sausages.

Nevertheless, there is still a shortage of suitable snack foods, especially for children. Most of those available tend to be high in sugar and also quite rich in fat.

Is the diet suitable for everyone?

NACNE does not recommend a specific diet, with absolute amounts of food, but a general restructuring of the current diet. As a result, such adjustments can be made in almost everyone's diet to make it healthier.

A word of caution is necessary, however, about people who have small appetites. As the NACNE-recommended diet contains more dietary fibre, it is likely to be more bulky than the traditional diet. In addition, the lower amount of fat and greater dependence on carbohydrate for energy also increase the volume of food to be eaten. Where the individual has a small appetite, insufficient amounts may be eaten to supply all of the nutritional needs. Thus the NACNE guidelines may require some modifications for children, the elderly and the sick.

Is it possible?

Since the publication of the NACNE report in 1983, considerable publicity has been given to healthy eating. Some critics of the report consider the measures as too severe for the British population, and therefore unrealistic. A recently published survey of British dietitians and their families has looked at how well such a motivated group has been approaching the dietary goals. It also asked them to change their diet for a week to comply with the dietary goals, if they were not already doing so. Results showed that the majority of the participants did manage to achieve the NACNE goals. The main obstacles that were reported included:

(1) Missing certain foods, such as sweets, snacks, chips, fat and dairy products.
(2) Extra time required in preparing basic foods.
(3) Lack of suitable foods available in the workplace and in restaurants.
(4) Lack of suitable snacks to eat between meals.
(5) Lack of convenience foods.
(6) The bulk of the diet.

The goal that was hardest to achieve was fat reduction, probably because so much food in the British diet contains hidden fat. The goal for dietary fibre increase was the next most difficult; goals for sugar, alcohol and salt were relatively

Table 11.3   Example of a target NACNE-style diet.

Meal	Menu
Breakfast	Wholegrain cereal (e.g. Weetabix); semi-skimmed milk Wholemeal toast with low-fat spread; low-sugar marmalade Coffee with semi-skimmed milk
Midmorning	Fresh orange; small packet peanuts or raisins Coffee with semi-skimmed milk
Lunch	Baked potato with cottage cheese filling *or* baked beans on wholemeal toast *or* wholemeal sandwiches, with ham or low-fat cheese
Midafternoon	Tea, with semi-skimmed milk; slice fruit cake
Dinner	Grilled.lean meat or fish *or* pasta dish, e.g. lasagne, perhaps made with vegetables rather than meat Jacket potato 2 or 3 vegetables, perhaps as salad Fresh fruit salad with yoghurt
Bedtime	Semi-skimmed milk drink Toast with low-fat spread

easily achieved. However, despite these reported difficulties, most of the participants in the study enjoyed their food more, or as much as usual, and were happy to continue with the new diet, along dietary guidelines proposed by NACNE. Some of the problems that were encountered were the result of changing suddenly to a new diet. These would not necessarily apply when people made changes gradually. Those subjects studied who were already achieving the dietary goals reported far fewer difficulties than those who changed to the NACNE-style diet overnight.

In conclusion there is no reason why a NACNE-style diet should not be adopted by the majority of the population, given sufficient information and motivation. Help from the government in terms of legislation on product composition and labelling, and from the food manufacturers in the form of more convenient 'healthy' food (and more healthy convenience food) is also necessary to achieve all the goals by the year 2000. Perhaps by then the typical diet of a Briton will be in line with that suggested in Table 11.3.

12
Food Habits and Food Choice

In order to consider the influences and determinants of food habits and food choice, it is important first to consider the meaning of these terms.

Food habits

Food habits are the typical behaviour of a particular group of people (or culture) in relation to food. They are integrated one with another, and each custom and practice has a part to play in the total approach to food. They are codes of conduct and may apply generally to a culture, or be a local variation on a general norm. They include food choice, as well as methods of eating, preparation, numbers of meals eaten per day, time of eating and the size of the portions eaten. Figure 12.1 summarizes some of the components of food habits.

Food habits are a product of the environmental influences on a culture; in general they are resistant to change. They are largely unconscious, since they are acquired at a young age from parents, and in this way the central food habits of a culture are transmitted from generation to generation.

The strongest influence on a child in its acquisition of food habits generally comes from the mother, who is usually the most closely involved with the provision of food. The child learns what is acceptable as food and what is not, often through reward and punishment. Food takes on an emotional significance from an

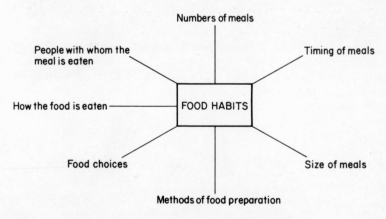

Fig. 12.1 Some components of an individual's food habits.

early age; this may override its nutritional value. An example of this is the use of sweets as rewards, gifts and tokens of affection. Problems may arise later in life if sweet foods are banned by a weight-reducing diet; this may be equated with a loss of comfort and a means of punishment.

After the initial acquisition of food habits within the home environment, the child learns more aspects of food-related behaviour from other people, or institutions, outside the home, who provide a secondary socializing influence. A major force is the school, where behaviour can be learned from other children. In addition, the school environment may provide models of food behaviour, through its school meals provision, tuck shops, and the more formal teaching in lessons. All of these will broaden the child's view of food, and will contribute to his or her own food behaviour patterns.

Later still, other people may influence the food habits, as different views are encountered in a wider social circle. Foreign travel also provides experience of different cultural food habits.

Although resistant to change, food habits in a cultural group – as well as in the individual – do change. The impetus to change may come from within the culture. For example, as a result of a greater number of women going to work, some of the traditional cooked meals may be eaten less often, and more convenience food may be used. Another example is increased migration, bringing new ethnic groups into close contact and allowing a mixing of food habits to occur.

The media use a variety of marketing techniques in an effort to alter food habits, with varying degrees of success. Food habits may also be re-educated in a more formal way, if the need arises for a change to the eating pattern, for example with a special diet.

Food choice

This covers those aspects of food habits that are related to the actual selection of foods. Although this may at first sound very straightforward, there is a complex interplay of factors influencing food choice.

If educators wish to change the food habits of a group of people, they must be aware of the influences on the food choice of the members of the group. In this way the education and advice given will not contradict or offend existing principles.

There are many ways to study food choice; viewpoints may be anthropological, economic, physiological, administrative, political, food chemical, psychological or marketing, as well as nutritional. Some of these approaches are considered here in a nutritional study of food choice.

There are two broad issues to consider in looking at the food choices made by an individual. These are the questions of availability of the food and of its acceptability to the consumer.

Availability

The factors determining availability of food are summarized in Table 12.1.

Physical factors

These include such issues as whether the food is locally grown or has to be transported to the area. For locally grown food, considerations include the suitability of

Table 12.1 Factors influencing availability of foods for determination of food choice.

Physical factors	Legislative factors	Economic	Food handling
Locality (soil/climate)	National/	Money available	Access to shops
Transport/marketing	international	Budget priorities	Cooking skills
Distribution costs	laws	Cost of foods	Knowledge
Perishability	Health	Significance of	Cooking facilities
	recommendations	foods	Time available
		Variety	

the soil and the climate. If the food is transported to the area, there must be an effective means of transport – by road, rail, air or sea. Isolated communities have a problem with the reliability of such supplies, especially if there are climatic extremes that prevent access at certain times of the year. Transportation from a long distance is likely to increase the price, so the food becomes excessively expensive.

Air transport has increased the availability of a wide variety of food around the world, whilst maintaining a reasonable price as long as demand is high.

Another constraint on food transport is its perishability. Fish are an excellent example. Many inland areas a long distance from the sea may never have salt-water fish, because of its rapid deterioration after being caught (they may have access to fresh-water fish, from local lakes or rivers). It is only when some form of preservation is used that transport of fish can become feasible.

Legislative factors

Government legislation aims to ensure that the food available for purchase is of a suitable standard and has not been adulterated in any way. Laws such as the Food and Drugs Acts and Consumer Protection Act provide various safeguards. The government may also dictate agricultural policy, not necessarily by directly telling farmers what to produce, but by regulating the prices received by the producers of the crops. Trades agreements or sanctions may operate between different countries.

Britain, as part of the European Economic Community, takes part in the Common Agricultural Policy, and thus operates various pricing and controlling practices within its framework. In addition, legislation throughout the EEC aims to standardize the composition of various manufactured products, especially in relation to permitted additives.

Most recently, pressure from health educators and the medical profession has increased the legislation on the labelling of foods, with information about their major nutrients and additives.

Economic factors

Within the range of foods available to them, people can only eat what they can afford, or choose to afford. This second point is important, since it brings into consideration the priorities which exist in spending money. On average, people in Britain spend about 20% of their budget on food, although those who are better off will spend a smaller proportion – and the poor will spend a higher proportion – of their overall budget on food. The actual *amount* of money spent will be greater among the wealthy than the poor.

Generally a higher-cost diet tends to be more varied, but also contains more fat and protein than a low-cost diet. People may see their food budget as one of the more flexible items in their expenditure; other expenses such as fuel, rent, cigarettes and alcohol may take priority.

When income is reduced and cutbacks are made in the food budget, these do not necessarily follow nutritional considerations and people do not always switch to a cheaper food of comparable nutritional quality. Other important considerations play a part. For example, the distribution of food within the family may change, with priority (especially for meat) being given to the father and any older children. Foods which have emotional significance will still be eaten, even though these may be more expensive. The tradition of the Sunday lunch, with a piece of meat as its centrepiece, is maintained for as long as possible. This emphasizes that food has a role other than simply providing nutrients.

Just as increasing wealth increases the variety of the diet, so a falling budget will reduce the variety. For a family living on a stringent food budget this makes sense. The mother (or primary carer) when shopping, knows exactly how much her purchases will cost and can therefore budget accordingly. In addition, as the foods are familiar, she can predict that the food will be eaten and not wasted.

Food handling

If food is available, and there is money with which to buy it, bringing it home and preparing it for eating remain as possible areas of difficulty. Getting to the shops and bringing food purchases home may be a major problem, especially for families with no transport, the old or disabled; it may affect the quantity and type of food bought, and the frequency of shopping. Access to larger shops (supermarkets) will generally mean that lower prices are paid than in smaller, local shops.

Modern technology is making this part of food availability easier. In some towns there are now computer links that allow customers to order food from a supermarket by telephone, and the food is later delivered to their home. Although this eases the problem of access, it does reduce the element of individual choice in the selection of a particular food item.

Once the food is in the kitchen, most of it has to be prepared in some way for eating. This depends largely on the knowledge and skill of the cook and the facilities available. Cooks' skills are variable, and in turn depend on personal experience of food and cooking, education, interest and, perhaps most importantly, time available for cooking.

This last factor has decreased considerably with increased female employment (over 50% of British women, and 2 out of 3 French women, are employed outside the home). This has been made possible by both the convenience food market, with many 'ready meals' available in the shops, and by many labour-saving appliances.

Acceptability

This is the second major area to consider in a study of food choice. The major factors involved are summarized in Table 12.2.

Table 12.2   Factors influencing acceptability of foods for determination of food choice.

Cultural	Physiological	Social/psychological
National identity	Physiological need	Status
Culture group	Hunger/satiety	of self
Core, secondary and peripheral foods	Appetite/aversion	of foods
	Sensory appeal	Group identity
Meal patterns	Personal preference/choice	Communication
Religious ideology	Therapeutic diets	Ritual
Taboos/prohibitions		Emotional support
		Reward, punishment

Cultural factors

Each cultural group around the world possesses its own typical food selection patterns. These may be quite similar to those of related cultural groups, but are unlikely to be the same.

In the United Kingdom there are regional differences in foods eaten, so that the Scots may be expected to appreciate haggis and other oat products, whereas the Welsh may be very fond of laver bread, which is a seaweed product. There are also similarities between the meal patterns of these two groups. For example, they probably both eat fish and chips, roast beef and rice pudding.

These traditional food choices associated with national identity represent security, a sense of belonging to a particular group. The strength and persistence of this national or cultural identity may be illustrated by two examples. Firstly, when people holiday in another country, many will seek out foods with which they are familiar. They may be prepared to try the local dishes, but out of curiosity, and often with a preconceived notion that they will be strange.

A more important example is that of migrants moving from one country to another. Migration from one's home country to settle permanently (or even for a finite, shorter period) in another country, brings with it a sense of alienation, or simply of difference from the adopted environment. At first integration involves those aspects of life visible to the outside world, such as the style of dress, or use of the host country's language. Food, however, is largely taken at home, and this is often one of the last aspects of the migrant's life to become even partly integrated.

Because it is a symbol of security and familiar to the migrant, food will provide a link with the homeland and a support in an alien environment. If in addition to providing a cultural identity, the food is also associated with religious beliefs and practices, traditional food habits may persist even longer. Studies on migrants into Britain show that traditional food practices persist strongly in first-generation migrants. In the second generation these practices are less widespread, unless they are associated with religious prescriptions, in which case adherence remains high. Conflict may arise between parents and children over the maintenance of traditional food habits, as the children are exposed more strongly to the host culture through school. The subject of immigrant foods and their nutritional implications in an alien culture are explored further in Chapter 14.

It is worth making a brief mention of 'temporary migrants', i.e. persons who live in another country for perhaps two or three years. Here again, an adherence to traditional food habits and a reluctance to include host-country foods in the diet are found. It appears that short-term migration does not bring with it the incentive to adopt new food habits in the way that permanent migration (albeit slowly) appears to do.

A person's culture will identify particular foods which fulfil specific roles in the overall eating pattern. The most important of these will be the *core foods*. These are the staple(s) around which the majority of meals are constructed. Without them, a meal would not be perceived as a meal. There are usually only a few core foods in any culture, sometimes only one. In the UK, bread (or cereal-based foods) and potatoes are considered to be core foods.

There are hazards inherent in over-reliance on a single core food. While the food is available, and if it is of a suitable nutritional quality, nutritional status can be maintained. If the crop should fail, either because of climatic changes, pest or disease damage, the absence of an alternative can have drastic results. This happened in the nineteenth century with the complete devastation of the Irish potato crop and subsequent famine. It also happens now, where local populations depend on a poor-quality staple food, such as yam or cassava and have no support crop, if the remaining land is devoted to production of crops for export (cash crops).

Secondary foods are defined as those that enhance the meal, but are not an essential part of it. They may be endowed with specific properties of their own. For example they may be seen as promoting strength (protein-rich foods such as meat), promoting good health (fruit and vegetables) or maintaining bodily forces in balance (by appropriate intake of 'hot' and 'cold' foods, as in some Asian cultures). They may also include foods which are seen as physiologically important for particular ages, or conditions of life. These might include such things as baby foods, 'invalid' foods, body-building foods, and foods to be eaten in pregnancy.

Thirdly, there is the category of *peripheral foods*. These encompass foods which are viewed as nonessential but pleasant extra items in the diet. Examples might include biscuits, confectionery, preserves, sauces, puddings, alcoholic beverages, luxury fruits. Also included in this group may be items which are viewed as 'prestige foods', generally by virtue of their rarity and/or cost. They are thus only eaten by a few people, or only on rare occasions, such as special festivals. Examples of such foods include Christmas pudding, Easter eggs, pumpkin pie. Foods with special properties may also come into this category: for example, special bedtime drinks, which are advertised as sleep-promoting.

Each national or cultural group has this repertoire of foods; whenever a meal is to be eaten, an appropriate choice is made from within these available foods. The choice will not be random, but will be a selection of items from each category, as is deemed fit by the culture. Table 12.3 shows how this might work in the UK.

Table 12.3   Core, secondary and peripheral foods in a typical British meal.

	Course 1 (savoury)	Course 2 (sweet)	Course 3 (sweet)
Core foods	Potato staple	Cereal staple (e.g. pastry)	Cereal staple (e.g. biscuit)
Secondary foods	Meat Vegetables	Fruit filling	
Peripheral foods	'Runny' liquid dressing (e.g. gravy)	Thick liquid dressing (e.g. custard)	Drink (e.g. tea)

Meal patterns. Many people in the West accept the pattern of three main meals a day as normal, but in some cultures, particularly poorer agricultural communities, only one meal might be eaten each day. The accompanying hunger attendant on this pattern of eating may be alleviated by the practice of chewing various leaves (such as coca or betel leaves), smoking cigarettes, drinking alcohol or even tea. This then becomes a food-related habit in itself. Longer periods of fasting may also be part of the cultural tradition, although they are more likely to be determined by religious prescription.

Taboos and prohibitions. As well as providing the norms for what may be eaten, cultural identity will also determine what should *not* be eaten. Each culture has clear ideas about what constitutes 'food' and what is 'non-food'.

Apart from general restriction on possible food items, more specific restrictions may exist for different sexes, or at particular stages of life. Many cultures have prohibitions associated with pregnancy, based on beliefs about possible effects on the foetus. Although generally without apparent foundation and normally harmless, some of these may restrict intakes of foods such as meat or other useful iron sources, for which needs are raised in pregnancy.

A very widespread taboo is that against cannibalism. Most cultures prohibit the eating of human flesh and most people would be revolted by the idea. However, even this deep-rooted taboo is not universal. There are records throughout history of individuals from societies where cannibalism is forbidden, actually eating their fellow humans in times of severe hardship. These have occurred in times of severe famine (as in Leningrad in 1941), and more recently where aircrash survivors have lived in inhospitable environments for long periods prior to rescue. These cases arouse considerable curiosity among observers and often induce a defensive attitude among those actually involved.

The world religions also proscribe the eating of particular foods, completely or at special times. These include taboos on pork among Moslems and Jews, and on beef among the Hindus. These are considered further in Chapter 14.

Physiological factors

The physiological need for food in man is modified by cultural, social and psychological influences and as such is often difficult to study.

Food is necessary to supply the appropriate amounts of energy for the maintenance of metabolism. Structural processes in the body also require a supply of fats, carbohydrates and proteins. To enable the body to utilize these macronutrients, it must be supplied with adequate vitamins and minerals.

The basic hunger drive causes people to eat. Sometimes it is refined into something more specific: an appetite for a particular food. There is some evidence from work on animals that such desires for particular foods are linked to a specific nutritional need. This is very difficult to demonstrate in humans and has therefore not been proven.

Appetite is associated with the memories of particular foods, especially with pleasurable memories. The opposite is an aversion to a specific food; this is likely to be linked to an unpleasant memory of that food, even if this is quite irrational to an outside observer.

Feelings of fullness (or satiety) at the end of a meal result in cessation of eating. The point at which satiety is reached does not have a very precise cut-off. With normal meals, the assessment of capacity is generally quite accurate. However, when the food is presented in a different manner, for instance as a large array of dishes, from which small amounts are eaten over a long period of time, satiety may never be reached. Alternatively, it is misjudged, and too much is eaten with resulting discomfort. A particularly attractive food may also cause overeating.

All foods stimulate the senses. The sensory role of food includes stimulation of the chemical senses of taste and smell, the visual sense and the sense of touch, by its texture and 'mouth feel'.

Chemical senses. The senses of taste and smell interact to provide information about the flavour of a food. Both taste and smell depend on specific receptors in the mouth and nose respectively. If either of these groups of receptors is unable to function, the perception of flavour is reduced, abnormal or absent. For example, most people will have experienced this in some degree when suffering from a cold.

The number of taste buds in the mouth is highest in children, who have them on the inside of the cheeks and throat, as well as over the surface of the tongue. From adolescence, only the taste buds on the tongue remain; these begin to decrease in later life, so that by the age of 70, there are only about a third the number of taste buds compared with a young adult. This reduces the ability to perceive tastes. Older people may remark that foods tasted better when they were young – there is a sound physiological basis for this.

Taste perception may also change in certain circumstances: pregnant women, patients after surgery and people suffering from cancer all report an altered ability to taste certain foods. Unusual appetites for particular foods may develop. If taste and smell are absent, or distorted, then enjoyment of food is diminished.

People are, however, prepared to eat and positively enjoy foods which they initially perceive as unpalatable. For example, the majority of people find beer, on first tasting, extremely bitter and not at all pleasant. However, as it is culturally a very acceptable food, this initial dislike is suppressed and a positive taste for beer is acquired. Other drinks for which a similar sequence appears to operate are coffee and tonic water (containing quinine). It is interesting that all three of these have a bitter taste, for which humans appear to have an initial aversion. In nature, many poisonous plants are bitter, and animals learn to avoid these. The aversion to the bitter taste is therefore an essential protective mechanism.

Visual sense. The appearance of the food is equally important. It contributes to the anticipation of a meal, and initiates the secretion of some of the digestive juices. It is especially important that food served to people with a poor appetite is presented in an attractive way. People are prepared to eat foods that look familiar, and are wary of the unfamiliar. It is very disconcerting to eat a meal blindfolded.

Appearance is so important to acceptance of a food that orange potatoes, brown peas or pink bread are likely to be rejected, however familiar their shape and smell. The food industry is well aware of the importance of the 'correct' visual stimulus, and uses a wide range of food colours to produce an acceptable finished product. There is currently a move to reduce the number of colour additives in foods, and return to the more natural appearance of the food.

Physical (textural) aspects. The feel of food in the mouth is the third aspect of its sensory role. This includes temperature, texture and any pain that the food may produce in the mouth. The temperature of a food is obviously an important aspect of its sensory appeal. Certain foods such as ice cream are expected to be cold, and others hot. If the food is presented at an unexpected temperature, either cold or hot, its appeal is reduced. Extremely cold foods may cause physical pain, as can very hot foods, which will burn the surfaces of the tongue and mouth linings. If a tooth has sensitive enamel or exposed dentine, extremely hot or cold foods can cause dental pain. Taste detection is reduced at cold temperatures, so food to be served cold requires additional flavouring. Thus, a spicy food served cold will appear to be less spicy than the same food served hot.

The texture of the food is also an important aspect of its sensory appeal. Food may be described in a variety of ways relating to the way it feels in the mouth: it may be crunchy, chewy, smooth, or 'melt in the mouth'. The fat content of a food enhances its mouth feel, contributing to a smooth texture, for example cream.

Some food constituents actually cause pain sensations in the mouth; the most notable of these is chilli. A chemical substance found in this spice irritates nerve endings in the mouth, triggering pain sensations.

Other substances cause a local anaesthetic effect; for example, chewing coca leaves, a widespread practice in parts of South America, numbs the senses in the mouth and reduces hunger. This is a custom often associated with infrequent meal patterns. In the UK, a slimming aid available in the form of a chewing gum similarly numbs the mouth, thereby reducing the physical appeal of any food that is eaten and hence (it is hoped) leading to weight loss.

Personal preference. Most people probably restrict their intake to those foods that they enjoy. New foods may be tried and become part of the routine diet, but there is a tendency for most diets to revolve around a relatively small number of different foods. Children are the age group most reluctant to diversify their diet. For some this range of foods can be so narrow that it is nutritionally risky.

It is, however, very important to the individual to be able to exercise some control over what is eaten. Loss of control over the choice of one's food intake can cause loss of appetite or problems of dietary noncompliance. The first of these may be a problem in institutionalized individuals, for example in a hospital, prison or residential home for the elderly. The catering staff might be unaware that the residents would like to exercise some choice. This is a particular problem where it is believed that the residents are not interested in food, so a monotonous menu cycle is used, with no choice for the diners. Introducing some choice into the menu restores a sense of self-determination over food and may well improve food intakes.

This has been the goal of the UK School Meals Service since 1980, with the introduction of a choice menu, including many cafeteria-style items, appealing to schoolchildren, in place of the traditional meal. As a result, uptake of the new-style school meals increased. The implications of these meals for health are discussed in Chapter 13.

In a different way, families existing on a low income have a restricted food choice for economic reasons. This may also lead to a low food intake due to lack of choice, loss of appetite and possible nutritional deficiencies.

The need to follow a special diet for ideological or therapeutic reasons will affect personal food selection and provides a further area where loss of control and self-determination may cause problems with compliance.

If a person is prescribed a weight-reducing diet, but does not recognize it as important, it will be seen as an infringement of their freedom of choice of food and may be ignored.

Children pose a particular problem in compliance with a therapeutic diet. If the food has to be different from that eaten by the rest of the family, it may be easier for the whole family to adopt the main aspects of the diet too. This prevents the child from feeling 'different'.

Special diets may be adopted for ideological reasons and these too impose constraints on the individual food choice. As these diets are usually embarked upon willingly, compliance with their requirements poses little problem. Some difficulties may again be encountered with children, whose parents attempt to impose the dietary restrictions. Problems of compliance may occur, especially away from home. In addition, the more restrictive diets may be nutritionally inadequate for the children.

Whatever the rationale, special diets constrain a person's freedom of choice. They make the person differ from his or her associates (this may be one of the objectives with certain ideologies). They may also create barriers to the sharing of food, causing alienation and possibly avoidance of social eating situations, or lack of compliance.

Giving as much freedom of choice as possible within the constraints of a therapeutic dietary regime will help to restore self-determination and promote compliance.

Social/psychological influences

Food choice is governed by other people's influences and the emotional response it may elicit, although the exact nature of this response depends on each person's experiences.

Status. Food and the way it is presented can be used to express status in a society. The most obvious distinction is that of having or not having food. It is generally assumed that the wealthy have plentiful access to food, while the poor are more likely to go hungry. In some societies, it is considered to be a sign of wealth or status to be obese.

Although food is generally perceived as a sign of status, individual foods and the way they are presented may enhance this. In Britain, high-status or prestige foods may include oysters, venison, grouse, asparagus and champagne. On the other hand, foods such as tripe, jellied eels and pig's trotters are equally unusual, but low-status foods. Everyday foods, because of their familiarity, also acquire relatively low status; these might include potatoes, baked beans, sausages and crisps. An elaborately prepared dish, with sauces and garnishes, is considered to be superior in status to plain cooked food. This may also be reflected in the attitude to the cook.

The perceived status of particular foods or combinations of dishes will dictate what is eaten in particular circumstances. When alone, it may not matter what we eat from the social point of view. Indeed, many people will confess to eating apparently bizarre combinations of food in these circumstances.

As soon as food is eaten in company, value judgements are made on the basis of the foods eaten. Choosing to serve very low-status foods may imply that the diners are seen as of low status. To create a good impression, higher status food is likely to be offered, prepared in a more elaborate way. Thus, the type of food shared at a meal implies more than the simple satisfaction of a physiological need.

Sharing food with others is in many ways a very symbolic gesture, reinforcing previously established links and confirming a sense of mutual identity. There is powerful peer pressure in food selection.

Foods do not necessarily possess the same status level for all time. Traditionally, white, refined wheat flour was expensive, and the white bread made from it was considered a luxury item. It therefore acquired high status. As milling became mechanized and the price of white flour fell, white bread came within the reach of all. In recent years, the health advantages of wholemeal bread have been recognized; as it is more expensive than white bread and therefore more readily affordable by the well-off, it has now become the high-status bread.

Communication. In addition to signalling messages about perceived status, food is also used as a more explicit means of communication. In western societies, a box of chocolates given as a present is perhaps the most widely used example of food acting as a token of affection. It may in some circumstances be easier to give the chocolates than to say what is actually felt. Similarly, in a difficult social situation, the British traditionally offer a cup of tea.

A family sitting down to a meal together are affirming their family identity. It is also a sign of caring and love from the provider of the meal. Rejecting the meal in this sort of setting has implications that reach beyond the unwillingness to eat the food, and may imply the rejection of the love offered, and isolation from the family unit.

Children often exchange small food items such as sweets to communicate their friendship. By rejecting this exchange they may emphasize their separateness. Reciprocal invitations to meals or parties are given by both adults and children; this ensures that friendships are maintained and do not disintegrate in the pressures of present-day existence.

Ritual. A special form of communication by means of food exists in the ritual use of food. Many religions use foods as offerings to their gods. Christians use bread and wine as ritual foods. The end of the peak growing season in most communities is marked by some form of ritual thanksgiving for the harvest, with the crops being offered as gifts, often to the poorest members of the community. In this way everyone can benefit at a time of plenty.

A further instance of the symbolic use of food occurs at Easter. This festival occurs in the spring, so even in societies where Easter is not celebrated, some form of 'rebirth' festival usually occurs. Lambs, chicks and eggs are frequently encountered as symbols of this rebirth.

Emotional support. Food represents security, so that in times of stress it can form an important support. This is believed to stem from the emotional security of infancy being linked with the providing of food. A sound basis here may well provide security about responses to food, for the rest of life.

Anxiety can provoke eating: at times of stress people may eat as a means of coping with tension. Such problems may result in prolonged overeating, causing overweight. The resultant concern about the excess weight may in turn cause further overeating.

Anxiety may also lead to feeding others: anxious mothers may overfeed their children, to relieve their own anxiety about them.

Abnormal eating patterns have also been associated with anxiety about one's role or position in society. It has been suggested that both overweight and anorexia nervosa may originate from a dissociation between the socially desired body size and that at which the individual feels psychologically at ease.

In the case of obesity, it is argued that overeating occurs as a deliberate attempt to add substance to the body (generally female), in an attempt to cope with the demands of the world. The converse is claimed to occur in anorexia nervosa, where the body size is deliberately reduced to escape from the pressures of society on the female.

13
Nutrition in Special Age Groups

Infants

Infants are totally dependent on other people for their food supply. In addition, the infant is growing rapidly and, for its age and size, has very high nutrient needs. Neither of these conditions normally occur again in a healthy individual.

The main aim of infant feeding is to satisfy nutritional needs in the best possible way, and to achieve a healthy infant who is growing and developing normally. Although the main concern here is with the principles of feeding normal infants, it must be remembered that infants who are ill, premature, handicapped, or in any other way outside the 'normal' category, can also be fed successfully, often by only minor adjustments of the normal practices.

Growth

Babies grow faster in the early months and more slowly in the latter part of the first year of life. The average baby in the West weighs 3.5 kg at birth; it will gain about 3.5 kg in the first 4 to 5 months and a further 3.5 kg in the remainder of its first year. Standard growth curves (see Fig. 1.3, p. 14) are used to monitor a child's development in terms of height and weight; deviations over a period of time from the child's usual curve may indicate faulty nutrition. Other causes may include illness, emotional problems or various other factors.

A child whose growth has deviated from the predicted curve is likely to show 'catch up' or 'lag down' growth rates, once the cause has been rectified.

Food for the infant

An infant at birth is able to suck, but not bite or chew pieces of food, so that its diet of necessity is a liquid one. The liquid designed by nature as food for the newborn is milk produced by its mother, providing not only nourishment but also immunological protection.

Alternative milks can be fed to infants: usually these have to be modified or fortified to make them nutritionally more suitable. The most widely used of these is that based on cow's milk. Modified soya milks are also available for infants who are not breast fed and who are allergic to cow's milk.

From about the end of the third month the baby can cope with a biscuit, rusk or cereal mixed with milk, by sucking and swallowing it with saliva. The ability to bite and chew lumps of food begins at 5 to 6 months, and it is at this stage that an increasing variety of tastes and textures can begin to be introduced into the baby's diet. An ability to chew lumpy foods by 6 or 7 months is an important developmental step and chewing is best learned at this age. If it is delayed, the child may have difficulty in learning to chew later. Ability to chew is also linked with early speech development. Thus early feeding is an important preparation for verbal communication.

By the age of 1 year, the infant has progressed from a newborn only able to suck liquids from a nipple or teat, to a 1-year-old attempting to feed itself. By this age, a child may have up to 8 teeth which help in the biting and tearing of food. Molar teeth for proper grinding of food develop late in the second year, when chewing ability becomes more fully developed.

In early infancy some of the digestive enzymes are not fully developed, so that the baby's tolerance of certain dietary components may be limited. The pancreatic juice secreted into the duodenum contains only a little lipase, the fat-digesting enzyme, during the first 3 months, implying a low fat-digesting capacity at this time. There are also very small amounts of pancreatic amylase for the digestion of starch before 6 to 12 months.

A small infant has the ability to absorb some undigested protein. This is of particular advantage for the absorption of antibodies, present in maternal milk. However, it may also result in the absorption of proteins such as egg albumen, or lactoglobulin from cow's milk, which may then set up an allergic response; these should be avoided for as long as possible.

Nutritional needs

Most of the information that exists about the nutritional needs of infants is based on observation of the intakes of healthy, normally growing, breast-fed infants. It must however be remembered that these figures are averages, and there is considerable variation between infants. The requirements of an infant in the first year of life are given in Table 13.1, and in Table 13.3 on p. 151.

Table 13.1   Recommended daily amounts for energy and protein for infants. From: DHSS (1979) *Recommended Daily Amounts of Food Energy and Nutrients for Groups of People in the United Kingdom (Report 15)*. London: HMSO.

Age range (months)	Body weight (kg) Boys	Girls	Energy (MJ) Boys	Girls	Protein (g) Boys	Girls
0–3	4.6	4.4	2.2	2.1	13	12.5
3–6	7.1	6.6	3.0	2.8	18	17
6–9	8.8	8.2	3.7	3.4	22	20
9–12	9.8	9.0	4.1	3.8	24.5	23

Energy. Energy needs are determined primarily by body size and composition, physical activity and the rate of growth. Infants have a high basal metabolic rate due to the large proportion of metabolically active tissue and the large loss of body heat over the relatively great surface area. As the child gets older, the energy requirement per unit of body weight decreases, although the total need for energy per child increases. The BMR accounts for approximately half of this energy need; the remainder is used largely to sustain growth in the young infant. By the age of 1 year, activity is using an increasing proportion of the total, and the energy used in growth may only represent one-quarter of the total.

Protein. Protein can be a source of energy, but in infants its role is almost entirely to support growth. Two amino acids, histidine and taurine, are essential in the infant's diet, in addition to the eight recognized as such for adults (see Chapter 6).

It is important that sufficient energy is provided in the infant's feed to allow the utilization of protein for growth. Excessive amounts of protein are undesirable and may be harmful in infants, as they increase the amounts of waste materials to be excreted in the urine. These remove water with them and might result in dehydration.

Fats. It is difficult to say how much fat an infant needs. In breast milk, fat provides 50% of the energy. Excessive amounts of fat (more than 3 to 4 g per kg of body weight) will result in reduced absorption and fat will appear in the faeces. This will also remove some calcium, thereby reducing calcium absorption. In addition, it is important that the milk contains sufficient amounts of the essential fatty acids; human milk provides about 1% of the total energy in the form of these fatty acids.

Carbohydrates. Carbohydrates supply 40 to 50% of the energy in an infant's diet. The predominant carbohydrate is lactose, which is broken down to glucose and galactose on digestion. Galactose is used in the development of the brain and nervous system in infancy. Babies have a limited ability to digest starch, as mentioned earlier. Apart from lactose, however, they can digest sucrose and utilize glucose. Excessive intakes of carbohydrate with insufficient fat may result in obesity.

Fluid. Because of a relatively small, total body water content, babies have a vital need for fluids. Their small size makes them susceptible to dehydration in very hot weather, or in illness.

At birth, 75% of the infant's body is water; this decreases to 69% at 1 year. Water is lost by evaporation through the skin and respiratory tract, through sweating at high environmental temperatures and in the faeces and urine. The volume of urine is dependent on the fluid intake and on the amount of solutes to be excreted. An adult kidney can concentrate solutes and so reduce water loss, if the intake of fluid is low. A baby's kidneys lack the ability to do this for some time. Thus feeding a diet with a high 'solute load', in particular with high protein and sodium contents, results in an increased fluid loss at the kidney. Under normal circumstances, infants will obtain sufficient fluid (150 ml per kg body weight) from their normal milk intake. However, difficulties arise when:

(1) A baby is fed an improperly prepared artificial milk feed (too concentrated).
(2) Limited amounts of feed are taken during illness.
(3) Losses via other routes are greater than normal, as in vomiting and diarrhoea, or in hot weather.
(4) The baby is fed solids at a very young age, without additional fluids.

In all of these cases, additional water should be given to prevent dehydration.

Minerals. Babies need a wide range of minerals in their diet. In particular, these include calcium and phosphorus for development of the skeleton, iron after the first 3 to 4 months of life and a number of trace elements such as copper, zinc, iodine, fluoride, cobalt, manganese and magnesium. All of these are provided in appropriate amounts for a normal infant in breast milk. Modified milk for infant feeding usually contains higher amounts of these than breast milk.

Calcium and phosphorus are used in the synthesis and remodelling of the skeleton and are present in teeth, which although not visible are present in infants within the gums. Calcium also plays a role in cell membranes as an enzyme activator, catalyses the blood clotting mechanism and regulates muscle contraction. Phosphate is necessary in all cells of the body for energy release and as a constituent of many enzymes. Excessive phosphate intake in early life may result in dangerously low serum calcium levels (hypocalcaemia) with tetany (muscular spasms). This occurs because the infant's kidneys do not excrete the excess phosphate, so blood levels rise and there is a compensatory fall in serum calcium. This is more likely to occur in formula-fed infants, or in those receiving alternative foods (such as unmodified soya products), or with excessively early weaning.

The initial iron reserves present at birth are used to maintain red cell production, but start to become inadequate from 4 to 6 months. Human milk is a poor source of iron; formula milks contain additional iron. It has, however, been estimated that up to 70% of the iron from human milk is absorbed by the infant, but only 10% of that from formula milk. The importance of introducing foods rich in iron early in weaning should be stressed. Without additional iron, babies are likely to become deficient, and their development will be slowed.

Breast milk supplies a wide range of minerals. In general absorption is higher from this source than from a comparable level of the mineral in formula milk.

Vitamins. Both human and cow's milk supply all of the vitamins required by infants in reasonably large amounts, with the exception of vitamin D. Recommended intake levels for the vitamins are based on their content in human milk, with the exception of vitamin D. This vitamin appears to be present in human milk in amounts smaller than those recommended. It is therefore desirable that a vitamin D supplement is given, if a child is not exposed to sunlight and during the winter months, to ensure adequate vitamin D levels, and consequently normal growth.

Meeting nutritional needs

A baby is most likely to be fed by breast milk or with a modified milk, most usually based on cow's milk, although unmodified animal milks may be used in some isolated communities.

The production of modified (formula) milks has progressed considerably from the time when 'modified' simply meant diluted, with possible sugar added. Many different modified milks are now produced. In the UK these may be classified into three categories, as shown in Table 13.2.

The formulae available in the UK comply with the guidelines for artificial feeds for infants; they should be reconstituted with the addition only of water in a given proportion to the quantity of powder used.

In many poor countries of the world the use of infant formulae has increased health problems, rather than solving or alleviating them. Where standards of hygiene are poor, with inadequate water supplies and nonexistent or poor sanitary facilities, it is almost impossible to prepare artificial feeds with the degree of cleanliness necessary to prevent infection. In addition, poverty may tempt the mother to prepare excessively dilute feeds, in an attempt to extend the supply of milk powder. This can lead to serious malnutrition in the infant. In such a situation, the only safe way of infant feeding is with human milk from the breast.

Table 13.2 Categories of infant milk formulae available in the United Kingdom. (*Note*: All of the milks contain added minerals, including iron and vitamins A, C and D. In some, trace elements may be added.)

Category	Protein	Fat	Carbohydrates	Minerals
Type 1: Cow's milk with added carbohydrate	Unmodified cow's milk protein; lower content	Cow's milk fat pattern; lower content	Lactose or maltodextrins added	Cow's milk pattern; lower content
Type 2: Skimmed milk with added fats and carbohydrate	Cow's milk protein; lower content	Vegetable and animal fats added; content approaches human pattern	Lactose or maltodextrin or starch added	Cow's milk pattern; lower content
Type 3: Skimmed milk with demineralized whey and mixed fats	Similar to human pattern	Animal and vegetable fats added; approaches human pattern	Lactose added	Low levels; similar to human milk

In more prosperous countries, many infants are successfully fed with infant formula. Several conditions should exist for successful bottle-feeding to occur:

(1) The family income should be adequate to buy formula in sufficient amounts.

(2) The standards of hygiene and facilities available should be sufficient to prepare the milk safely.

(3) The mother (or carer) should be adequately informed about the techniques involved and should be able to follow them.

Breast feeding or bottle feeding?

Breast feeding is the ideal method of feeding for most infants, with the exception of a few unusual situations. These may include a mother taking drugs that may be harmful to the baby, a very premature baby, or one with malformations making normal feeding impossible. In addition to the nutritional advantages of human milk to the infant, there are also immunological and possible long-term health benefits.

Nutritional benefits

As recommended intakes for infants are usually based on data from breast-fed babies, it follows that nutritionally, breast milk comes close to recommended intake levels. The composition of breast milk is not constant, with the most rapid change occurring during the first week of lactation. There is variation between mothers, and also during a feed, with the milk secreted towards the end of a feed (hind milk) being richer in fat and therefore higher in energy value than the fore milk, at the start of the feed. It has been suggested that this may play a part in appetite control, with the richer hind milk providing a feeling of satiety.

This mechanism cannot occur with a bottle-fed baby, whose feed is of the same concentration throughout.

Proteins. The proteins found in breast milk are predominantly whey proteins, including alpha-lactalbumin, serum albumin, lactoferrin and various immuno-globulins; casein forms a small proportion (30 to 40%) of the total protein. In unmodified cow's milk, approximately 80% of the total protein is casein, and whey proteins are in the minority. Additionally, cow's milk contains beta-lactoglobulin, which is believed to be its major allergenic component. The casein from cow's milk forms tough and leathery curds in the stomach, which are more difficult to digest than the softer, flocculent curds from breast milk casein. Further, breast milk contains amino acids that are essential in young infants who cannot synthesize them at this age. Although cystine is present in formula milks, taurine may be absent.

Carbohydrates. Lactose concentrations in breast milk are greater than those in unmodified milks. Formula milks contain additional carbohydrate in the form of starch, maltodextrins or lactose, but the starch-containing milks should be restricted to the older infant. Lactose increases the acidity of the faeces, which is thought to be important in suppressing the growth of *Escherichia coli* in the intestines of breast-fed infants, thus reducing the risk of gastroenteritis. Moreover, lactose enhances the absorption of calcium, explaining the better absorption rates of this mineral from human milk.

Fats. Although the total fat contents of human and cow's milks are similar, the fatty acid contents differ. The short-chain fatty acids present in cow's milk are absent from human milk. Human milk is richer in polyunsaturated fatty acids, in particular linoleic acid, one of the essential fatty acids.

Fats from human milk are more efficiently absorbed than fats from cow's milk. This is attributed to the presence of a lipase in breast milk, which begins the digestion of fat before pancreatic enzymes are secreted.

Human milk is higher in cholesterol content than formula milks. The significance of this is unknown. It has been suggested that a high cholesterol intake in early life may prime enzyme systems, to cope more effectively with cholesterol intakes in later years. However, at present there is no evidence to support this theory.

Vitamins. Most vitamins, with the exception of vitamin C, nicotinic acid and folate, are found in smaller amounts in human milk than cow's milk. However, these amounts are assumed to be appropriate for the baby. Some vitamins in human milk vary with maternal dietary intake: this includes vitamin A, thiamine, riboflavin, folate, vitamin B_{12} and vitamin C. In recent years a water-soluble vitamin D sulphate fraction has been identified. This may provide further vitamin D activity in human milk, although the exact nature of this remains unclear. Human milk is also believed to contain certain binding factors for folate and vitamin B_{12}, which may facilitate their absorption.

Minerals. Breast milk contains less calcium, phosphorus, potassium and sodium than cow's milk, but more copper, iron, cobalt and selenium. In the production of infant formula, many of these mineral levels are modified to make the pattern resemble that of human milk more closely. The occurrence of hypertonic dehydration and hypocalcaemic tetany has declined recently in the West, with the introduction of low-solute modified milks.

Iron is added to milk formula during its manufacture, making the level in formula higher than that in breast milk. Nevertheless, the small amount of iron present in human milk is sufficient, as it is better absorbed. This is attributed to various iron-binding substances in human milk, which increase its availability for absorption. At the same time, little iron remains available for bacterial growth in the gut, reducing the risks of gastroenteritis. Similar binding factors are believed to increase absorption of zinc from human milk.

Guidelines exist for the composition of formula milks that are based on the nutrient contents in human milk. However, some nutrients are present in greater amounts in formula milk, in an effort to compensate for their poorer availability from this source. As a result, and within the limits of current knowledge, artificial milks contain nutrients in amounts suitable for infant feeding.

Immunological benefits

The anti-infective and protective properties of human milk are derived from the presence of specific anti-infective substances and white blood cells. An extremely high concentration of these protective factors is found in colostrum, which is produced in the first few days after birth. The main protective substance is secretory immunoglobulin A (IgA). IgA is known to protect the mucosal surface of the gut, acting as a barrier against many infective organisms. IgA from human colostrum has been said to fill the 'immunity gap' for a newborn infant, until its own immune system can begin to provide protection. The white blood cells and these immunoglobulins provide protection against many common bacteria, such as staphylococci, streptococci, pneumococci, salmonellae and *Escherichia coli* (*E. coli* is a major cause of gastroenteritis). Other factors contributing to the overall immunological benefit of breast milk include lysozyme (from the white blood cells), complement and lactoferrin.

Many studies in various countries have demonstrated a lower incidence of infections in breast-fed infants, with an associated lower mortality. In the West most of these infections can be treated successfully, although some do end in death. In developing countries, the increased vulnerability to infection of a bottle-fed baby makes death rates considerably higher.

Breast feeding ensures a delayed exposure to cow's milk and therefore reduces the risk of developing an allergy to cow's milk proteins. These are completely foreign to man and can result in various allergic manifestations including eczema, rhinitis (runny nose), asthma and intestinal inflammation. Where possible it is advisable to breast feed any baby where there is a risk of allergy, for example if the parents or any siblings exhibit allergic tendencies.

Future health benefits

It has been claimed that breast feeding confers advantages in terms of the later health of the baby. These advantages include less obesity, heart disease and multiple sclerosis, as well as better dental health. However, evidence to substantiate these claims is very difficult to obtain.

Weaning

The process of weaning an infant marks the transition from an exclusively milk diet to one containing predominantly solid foods. The age at which this occurs varies between different cultures and communities, from as early as 2 months to the end of the infant's first year. Neither of these extremes is nutritionally ideal. The optimal age at weaning should be between 4 and 6 months.

From about 4 months, a milk diet alone starts to become incapable of meeting the needs for iron. Failure to introduce solids by 6 months may, in addition, lead to an inadequate intake of energy. Excessively early weaning is however to be avoided, and if signs of hunger are appearing in a child below about 3 months, milk intake should be increased in preference to solids.

Early weaning may result in a fat baby, or trigger allergies to common foods such as egg white, wheat flour and cow's milk, if these are introduced at a time when the digestive tract can still absorb whole proteins. There is also a risk of overloading the digestive system, whose enzymes may not be fully functional, or the excretory system, where the ability to concentrate urine is still undeveloped.

In many parts of the world, the first weaning food to be introduced is usually a cereal. In the West, it may be a specially formulated cereal, designed for weaning and enriched with a number of nutrients. In developing countries the cereal is usually the local staple, prepared as a gruel or porridge.

As the child becomes accustomed to the novelty of solid foods, the next to be introduced are usually fruit and vegetables, which may be cooked and puréed or sieved. After these, minced meat, fish and other sources of protein, such as sieved soft cheese or egg yolk, can be added.

As chewing ability develops, the pieces of food offered should become more distinct, allowing chewing to be practised. Pieces of food to be held in the hand for biting and chewing are very useful. By the age of 1 year a child should have completed the process of weaning.

The two major objectives of weaning are:

(1) To supply all the nutrients needed by the infant in a nutrient-dense form. In particular attention should be paid to energy, protein, iron, vitamin C and vitamin D.

(2) To train the palate and guide it towards a healthy food choice in the future.

The toddler and pre-school child

The years between 1 and 5 represent a consolidation of early food habits and the development of some independence in relation to food. Growth is generally slower than in the first year of life, but it tends to occur in spurts, often accompanied by surges of appetite. Activity also increases markedly during the second year of life, as the child becomes increasingly mobile. Development of a full dentition by about the age of 2 years also increases the range of foods that can safely be eaten.

Because capacity remains relatively small, one between-meal snack may be needed between each of the three main meals of the day. It is important to keep healthy eating guidelines in mind when selecting snack foods. These can include fresh or dried fruit, wholemeal sandwiches, raw vegetables as 'finger food' to chew, dry breakfast cereals and low-sugar or savoury biscuits. Meals should consist of nutrient-dense foods, with at least 250 ml of milk (or alternatives) daily, and cereals or bread used to fill up to appetite. Appetite remains the best guide to overall food needs at this age.

Food refusal can be a major problem, particularly in the second year; experimenting with food, usually in the form of bizarre dietary mixtures, is a more common practice among 4-year-olds, having been reported in up to 30%.

School-age children

Pre-adolescent (5–11 years)

When children start school their eating patterns begin to be influenced by factors other than the home environment.

Growth rate is relatively slow during these years but still occurs nonlinearly, with surges accompanied by increases of appetite.

Apart from growth, activity is the other major influence on appetite in this age group. Starting school may significantly alter a child's activity pattern; the direction of the change depends on how active the child was during the pre-school years.

School may be emotionally taxing for children which may be reflected in their food intake. A child who has mixed with relatively few children before starting school may contract a number of 'childhood illnesses' which will take a toll on his or her appetite, adding up to an inadequate food intake over a number of months. A study of schoolchildren in Glasgow has shown that morbidity, especially from diarrhoeal illness, does reduce growth.

School meals

For many children, school meals are a major influence on food intake. In the UK prior to 1980, the local education authorities (LEA) were obliged by law to provide a midday meal for schoolchildren that satisfied certain nutritional criteria. Broadly, these involved meeting one-third of the daily recommended intake for energy and 40% of the recommended amount of protein, with specifications as to the sources of the protein, and the foods which were to be used. After the abolition of this legislation, radical changes have occurred in the British school meals system, with cash cafeteria systems in many senior schools, offering a choice of foods to their pupils. The younger children in school may have a more limited choice, perhaps selecting from two main meal items, vegetables and puddings. The amount of waste collected at the end of meals is now much less. There is also an opportunity for children to make decisions about their own food. This can be of positive benefit where the provision of the meal is linked to a nutrition education programme, informing the children about healthy eating and the foods to choose for a healthy diet.

Concern has been expressed that the free choice in cash cafeteria systems allows children to select nutritionally unbalanced meals. Yet a comparison of traditional school meals and self-selected cash cafeteria meals found that both provided at least 33% of the recommended daily allowance for energy. Fat content was however shown to be higher in the latter and there was a trend to a higher sugar content.

Evidence from the 1986 DHSS study of the diets of British schoolchildren showed that school meals compared reasonably well with other sources of lunch-time food, such as cafés and take-away outlets. Fat content of these meals supplied 39 to 45% of the energy; meals from home provided 37 to 38% of energy as fat. The children having meals in cafés or take-away outlets also had lower lunchtime intakes of protein, iron, calcium, retinol, thiamine, riboflavin and vitamin D. In all these respects, school meals were better nutritional value.

A survey by the National Dairy Council in 1981 showed that overall, 46% of children had school lunch, although this figure was higher in the 5 to 10-year-olds (52%), than in the 14 to 18-year-olds (38%).

In a survey in London in 1984, 7% of the schoolchildren sampled claimed they could not eat the meal provided for religious reasons. In many towns and cities where there are ethnic minority groups, some provision may be made within the school meals service, although this becomes more difficult when numbers of children are small. However, this illustrates very well the new food experiences to which children may be exposed on coming to school.

There is some debate about the role of the school meal in nutrition education. Some see it as an essential, practical illustration of good nutritional principles. However, it is also argued that the school meal should be separate from the educational atmosphere in the school and provide a break from learning for the pupils. It seems inevitable, however, that if children have lunch in school, they will begin to learn about other foods that they may have never encountered before and will acquire attitudes to eating from their peers.

Nutritional needs

Recommended intake figures for children give values for all of the major nutrients (Table 13.3). It should be remembered, however, that with the exception of the recommendations for energy, these figures represent sufficient to cover the needs of 95% of all children. Therefore an individual child may be perfectly adequately nourished, taking in a much lower level of a specific nutrient than is actually quoted.

The recommended figures for energy represent the average of the actual requirements for children in each age group, as explained in Chapter 9. Appetite is generally considered the best guide to energy needs.

Composition of the diet. This should be similar to that of a normal, healthful diet, as described in Chapter 11. The NACNE report had reservations about the application of its dietary guidelines in children below the age of 5 years, but not after this age. The goals therefore should be to provide a varied mixture of foods, to include whole cereals, pulses, fresh vegetables and fruit, together with moderate amounts of lean carcase meat, poultry, fish and lower-fat dairy foods. Sugar intake should be limited, preferably being obtained from natural, whole sources of sugar, such as fruit (fresh or dried), rather than refined sugar products. If refined sugar is included, it should form part of a meal, and be avoided as a snack food.

Sweet eating by children is an almost universal practice in the West. A study of young adolescents (11–12 years) in 1984 in the UK found that 20% of their energy was derived from sugars. Many children consume sweets daily, and at intervals throughout the day. This can have several detrimental effects. Most notably, a frequent intake of sugar, particularly in a sticky form, is a major cause of tooth decay.

Table 13.3 Recommended daily amounts of food energy and some nutrients for children and adolescents in the United Kingdom. From: DHSS (1979). *Report 15.* London: HMSO.

Age (yrs)	Energy (MJ)	Protein (g)	Thiamine (mg)	Riboflavin (mg)	Nicotinic acid (mg)	Ascorbic acid (mg)	Vitamin A (µg)	Vitamin D (µg)	Calcium (mg)	Iron (mg)
Boys										
Under 1	See Table 13.1	See Table 13.1	0.3	0.4	5	20	450	7.5	600	6
1	5.0	30	0.5	0.6	7	20	300	10	600	7
2	5.75	35	0.6	0.7	8	20	300	10	600	7
3–4	6.5	39	0.6	0.8	9	20	300	10	600	8
5–6	7.25	43	0.7	0.9	10	20	300	a	600	10
7–8	8.25	49	0.8	1.0	11	20	400	a	600	10
9–11	9.5	57	0.9	1.2	14	25	575	a	700	12
12–14	11.0	66	1.1	1.4	16	25	725	a	700	12
15–17	12.0	72	1.2	1.7	19	30	750	a	600	12
Girls										
Under 1	See Table 13.1	See Table 13.1	0.3	0.4	5	20	450	7.5	600	6
1	4.5	27	0.4	0.6	7	20	300	10	600	7
2	5.5	32	0.5	0.7	8	20	300	10	600	7
3–4	6.25	37	0.6	0.8	9	20	300	10	600	8
5–6	7.0	42	0.7	0.9	10	20	300	a	600	10
7–8	8.0	47	0.8	1.0	11	20	400	a	600	10
9–11	8.5	51	0.8	1.2	14	25	575	a	700	12b
12–14	9.0	53	0.9	1.4	16	25	725	a	700	12b
15–17	9.0	53	0.9	1.7	19	30	750	a	600	12b

a = No intake is necessary where there is sufficient exposure to sunlight; supplements may be needed in winter.
b = Girls with heavy menstrual losses may have a higher need.

This is discussed more fully in Chapter 16. The NACNE report recommends that no more than 10 kg of sugar per person per year is eaten in the form of between-meal snacks; this represents less than half of the current intake of such snacks.

A second effect is that of supplying 'empty energy'. Sweets are an excellent example of a food that is lacking in nutrients other than energy. As a result, the total daily energy need may be met, without accompanying nutrients. Not only do the sweets then reduce the appetite for further food intake; in addition they also increase the necessity for the remaining food intake to be highly nutrient-dense. If sweets are eaten in addition to a normal, adequate food intake, the extra energy will cause overweight. Most western parents (and their children) would consider not eating sweets at all to be unendurable. In this case most nutritionists and dentists would agree that the best way to eat a few sweets is perhaps as a once-a-week treat, after a meal, and all in one go. In this way most of the possible harmful effects are minimized.

Adolescents (11–18 years)

The adolescent years are a period of great physical and emotional change, marking the development of the child into an adult.

The physical changes occur over a relatively short period of time, usually about two years, and include gains, in boys, of some 20 cm in height and 15 to 20 kg in weight. Increases in girls are generally smaller. In addition, there are also changes in body composition: lean body mass increases by at least a factor of two (in girls) to three (in boys), body fat increases slightly in boys, but may increase threefold in girls. The increased skeletal size is accompanied by a higher calcium content. Food intake must change to supply the nutrients for these dramatic developments.

The nutritional requirements are given in Table 13.3 on p. 151, based on the recommended amount figures in DHSS *Report 15*.

The timing of the need for this increase depends on the individual; there is considerable variation in the exact age at which the pubertal growth spurt begins. In the West, peak appetite occurs around the age of 12 in girls and 14 in boys, apparently corresponding to the most rapid growth period. Nutrient needs increase both to meet the demand for new tissue synthesis: with calcium, phosphorus and vitamin D for bone or protein, zinc and iron for muscle, as well as to supply the energy for this synthesis (energy and B vitamins). If energy needs are not met, the growth spurt may be delayed or reduced. However, energy needs for growth probably do not exceed 10% of total energy requirements at this time.

In addition, there is an increased blood volume and, at puberty, menstruation begins in girls, further raising the need for iron. Once the rapid growth spurt is over, nutrient needs settle down to adult levels. The quality of the diet should be high during the whole adolescent period, but especially during the growth spurt.

In developing countries, the growth spurt occurs later than in the West and may also be slower, resulting in smaller adult stature. In well-fed societies, the link between socio-economic status and the size of the child is less obvious.

Attitudes to food and eating patterns

Many teenagers eat erratically, rather than at commonly accepted meal times. If little or nothing is eaten throughout most of the day, it becomes difficult to meet the whole day's needs in one meal. Conversely, there may be continuous snacking throughout the day; such an intake pattern increases vulnerability to nutritional inadequacy. If this pattern persists for a number of years, the individual may lose the ability to recognize hunger and satiety and be unable to decide when to start and stop eating. This chaotic eating is a major problem in certain disorders seen in western society. In the extreme, these take the form of bulimia nervosa (compulsive eating with purging or vomiting) and anorexia nervosa (compulsive fasting). They are described more fully in Chapter 3.

Social pressures to conform to the peer group are strongly reflected in the choice of food, both in school and in social settings.

Older teenagers may spend time in public houses drinking alcohol. This provides 'empty energy', but in addition may lead to the irresponsible use of alcohol in later years.

There is an increased tendency to miss meals in the home environment, so that possibly few well-balanced meals may be eaten. A study by the National Dairy Council in Britain in 1981, found that 20% of 14 to 18 year olds missed breakfast, but only 8% of younger children did so. Missing breakfast is more likely to result in nutritional inadequacy than missing lunch or the evening meal, as the latter may be replaced by snacks. Parental pressure to change any of these habits may meet with considerable resistance. However, parents can determine what foods are actually available in the house for the hungry teenager to eat. If the selection is of healthy, well-chosen foods, then that is what he or she will eat.

Some special problems

Vegetarianism. An increasingly common form of rebellion among teenagers is the rejection of the omnivorous diet of their parents, in favour of a vegetarian (non-meat) diet. The reasons for this choice may include compassion for animals; concern over western self-indulgence in food and exploitation of the world's poorer countries; a dislike of the taste, texture or smell of meat; peer pressure; or, simply, a desire for independence. Unfortunately many of these new vegetarians have an inadequate understanding of nutritional principles, so that the traditional 'meat and two vegetables' becomes just 'two vegetables', or baked beans on toast. There is often very little attempt to introduce other dietary items, such as pulses, cereals and grains, into the diet to replace the animal foods being avoided. In this way iron, nicotinic acid and zinc may become very inadequate.

Parents catering for a single vegetarian in the family may find menu planning troublesome.

Teenage athletes. Nutrition and sport is discussed more fully in Chapter 14. Teenage athletes are particularly vulnerable, having additional needs related to their growth. Most schoolchildren participate in some sport, which involves no more than 2 to 3 hours per week; playing in school teams may occupy a further 3 to 4 hours each week. This amount of extra physical activity increases nutritional needs slightly, but probably not beyond the limits of the usual recommended intakes for all nutrients, except energy. As with adult athletes, there is a particular need for carbohydrate, preferably in its starchy form, to sustain muscle glycogen levels. School team coaches should be aware of this need.

The most vulnerable group of teenage athletes are those who aspire to become top-class. This may involve 6 or more hours of training daily, from a very young age. This imposes a considerable nutritional need both for energy and associated nutrients in line with the energy increase. Where a normal, moderately active teenager may require 12.6 MJ per day, one in training might need an additional 8.4 to 12.6 MJ. This represents an enormous amount of food, which there may be little time to eat. Many teenage athletes may be reluctant to eat so much food, for fear of becoming overweight, or simply appearing greedy. Yet full athletic potential with normal growth cannot be achieved without the appropriate nutritional input.

Pregnant teenagers. The general principles of nutrition in pregnancy and associated problems are described in Chapter 14. Pregnant teenagers have additional needs, by virtue of both their age and the pregnancy.

Studies in many countries have shown that the risks of pregnancy complications, maternal mortality, stillbirth and low birth weight babies are increased in pregnancies where the mother is below 17 or above 35 years of age.

Many of the teenage pregnancies occur in single girls, which brings further social and emotional problems to compound the nutritional stress. If the pregnancy is unwanted, the girl may try to limit her weight gain and even lose weight to conceal it. There may be parental rejection and she may have to leave home; this reduces her opportunities of obtaining a healthy diet.

Attendance at antenatal clinics may be erratic or nonexistent, so helpful advice is missed. Many teenage girls may normally have a poor diet, lacking in iron, zinc and many vitamins. The additional needs of pregnancy may simply not be recognized, or if recognized, not met.

There will, however, be pregnant teenagers who will care for themselves in pregnancy. The girl's own body is still growing and developing (particularly in the younger adolescent). She must ensure that enough food is eaten to meet both her own needs and those of the developing baby. Failure to do so will compromise both her own health and that of the baby.

Dieting. It has been estimated that some 10% of adolescents are obese in the West, although exact figures are difficult to obtain. Obesity is more common among adolescents from lower income families. There is a greater degree of inactivity among the overweight, which probably contributes to its persistence, and is possibly its cause.

The incidence of dieting among adolescents is greater than 10%; it is most widespread among girls. Dieting is erratic: many use 'crash' diets, eating little for days and making little effort to balance the rest of the food intake. There is a danger that the dieting becomes a habit, establishing a chaotic eating pattern, or 'noneating' pattern. Adolescent girls tending towards thinness should be warned about the dangers of their food habits. A body mass index (see Chapter 3) of below 18 is a useful marker of the need for counselling.

Dieting is less of a problem among boys, although some cases of anorexia have been reported. In some of these there was an obsessional preoccupation with sport as a major means of weight control, rather than the more usual vomiting or purging seen in girls. Usually, however, adolescent boys are primarily concerned with becoming taller and stronger and concentrate more on body building. The routes to sound nutrition education for adolescents may well lie in concentrating on these disparate ambitions of male and female teenagers: muscle and height in males, and slimness in females.

Areas of nutritional concern. Despite all of the possible adverse influences described, most teenagers appear to be healthy, and grow and develop normally. They seem fit, are able to partake in sport and enjoy physical and mental well-being. Nevertheless, specific nutrients may be inadequate in some diets, including iron, calcium, riboflavin, vitamin A and vitamin C.

Iron intakes have been found to fall consistently below levels recommended both in the UK and USA. In the USA, prevalence of inadequate intakes was greatest among adolescents from the poorest sectors and among ethnic minority groups. The DHSS study of British schoolchildren in 1986 found average iron intakes of 10 to 11-year-old and 14 to 15-year-old boys and girls to be below recommended levels. These may be a particular problem among the older girls, who are dieting and also have heavy menstrual losses.

Calcium needs are high in adolescence. There is, however, no evidence that dietary calcium is limiting for bone growth at this time. However, poor calcium accretion into bone, with a consequently smaller final bone mass, may predispose to the earlier development of osteoporosis. Since calcium is primarily derived from dairy products, milk intake may be a good indicator of calcium status. It has also been suggested that milk intake is closely related to riboflavin status.

In addition, a relationship has been described between milk drinking and the selection of a nutritionally adequate diet. The DHSS survey mentioned above found calcium intakes to be within recommended levels. The lowest intakes were among the 14 to 15-year-old girls, whose riboflavin intakes were also below recommended levels.

Adolescents may rarely eat carotene-rich fruit and vegetables; liver, the main source of preformed retinol, is often quoted as the most disliked food by teenagers. In a USA survey, over a third of adolescents (10 to 16 years) had vitamin A intakes 50% below standard, with low serum vitamin A values. A British survey of young adolescents also found intakes to be below those recommended. It is impossible to assess the true extent of any possible vitamin A deficiency, due to a lack of standard values. There might also be some concern about excessive intakes from supplements used in sport and treatment of acne.

The pattern of snack eating among adolescents may increase their vulnerability to vitamin C deficiency. Fruit and vegetables, the main sources of the vitamin, may be almost completely absent from the diet. Nevertheless, the widespread eating of potatoes and potato products provides a moderate but consistent source of vitamin C, even when few other sources are eaten.

In general, there is an increasing concern that the roots of many diseases of middle and later life may lie in the childhood diet. There is much evidence that overweight, and a high fat, salt and sugar intake with little dietary fibre, are the main contributors to disease in later life. It is argued that more effort should be directed at adolescents, to establish more healthy eating patterns at this age, before early adulthood.

Young adults

At present the diet of many young adults also exhibits features of the adolescent diet, with meal skipping and generally low intakes. A survey by the Ministry of Agriculture, Fisheries and Food in Britain in 1986 looked at the diets of 15 to 25 year olds. Bridging the age range from adolescence to early adulthood, this survey was in a position to show if the eating habits of the teenager become more 'normal' as adulthood is reached.

The survey found that those still living with parents or who were married had more conventional food habits. Generally, women were found to be more food-conscious, being more concerned about weight, processed food and additives.

Nutrient intakes in general were low in some subgroups, especially the 15 to 18-year-old males and the 19 to 21-year-old women. Of these, lowest intakes occurred in those who were diet-conscious or living alone. Nutrients that were particularly low included energy (80% of recommended), iron (69%) and thiamine (92%). Both men and women living alone had low intakes of energy, fat, carbohydrate, dietary fibre, iron, and vitamin B_{12} in women only.

Thus the survey highlights a continuing vulnerability to poor dietary intake among older adolescents and young adults. The change to a more conventional and nutritionally adequate intake appears to come only on marriage, or in a stable sharing domestic arrangement.

The middle aged

Aging is a continuous process throughout life. The visible signs that are widely associated with aging first appear in most people in middle age. This term is used here to refer to the age band from approximately 45 to 60 years. It may be that by delaying or preventing the early stages of aging, better health may be achieved in the older years.

Certain aspects of the aging process start to become more apparent at this stage:

(1) Changes in body composition and physiological function.
(2) Increase in chronic diseases and disabilities.
(3) Changes in food intake patterns, with reduced food intake and possibly increased intake of alcohol.

Changes in lean body mass

Throughout adult life there is a progressive reduction in lean body mass and a compensatory accumulation of adipose tissue. As the lean body mass is metabolically very active, and the adipose tissue is not, there is a fall in metabolic rate with age. This is believed to be a major contributor to the increased prevalence of obesity seen in the West. Obesity prevalence increases steadily with age (see Table 13.4).

Table 13.4 The increase of overweight with age, in the UK (OPCS, 1984).

	20–24	25–29	Age in years 30–40	40–50	50–60	60–65
Men						
Overweight (Body mass index 25–30)	19%	26%	34%	43%	43%	44%
Obese (BMI above 30)	3%	3%	6%	9%	7%	10%
Women						
Overweight	16%	15%	21%	28%	32%	36%
Obese	5%	5%	6%	9%	14%	15%

Prevention of the onset of obesity is therefore important. Its main objectives should be a gradual reduction in the food intake, particularly the energy-dense fat component. In addition, and probably more importantly, there should be maintenance of or an increase in physical activity. This will be of benefit in several ways: by increasing energy output directly, slowing the loss of lean body mass and thus the fall in metabolic rate, and ultimately preventing obesity and its associated medical complications. In addition there will be benefits for bone health, as explained below.

Loss of bone density with age

One of the most widely studied age-related changes in body composition and function is that of the loss of bone density with age or *osteoporosis*.

This is believed to begin around the age of 40 years and to proceed initially at a relatively slow rate. There is a period of more rapid bone loss in women for the first 15 to 20 years after the menopause, related to the loss of the female hormones, particularly oestrogens. Post-menopausal women treated with oestrogen do not exhibit this rapid reduction in their bone density; there may, however, be clinical problems associated with long-term oestrogen therapy. In men, the loss of bone density is slow and consistent. There is considerable individual variation in the rate of loss. In many people, the progressive loss of bone density causes no clinical problems. In others the osteoporotic bone is sufficiently weak to fracture under even a minor impact. This poses a health problem in the elderly, particularly women, of whom 40% may have experienced such a fracture by the age of 70.

Current evidence suggests that it is desirable to achieve a high bone mass by the age of 20 to 30, to minimize the effects of later osteoporosis. Several factors may be involved in determining this bone mass:

(1) *Previous dietary intake.* Since the major components of 'lost' bone are protein and calcium, it is reasonable to assume that a higher initial content of these will be beneficial. Indeed, populations with a high calcium intake do maintain a higher bone density in old age. In America, a similar phenomenon apparently related to ethnic origin occurs among the black population, who have greater bone densities in early adult life and later suffer less osteoporosis. An increased protein intake, however, causes increased urinary loss of calcium, and so reduces the amount retained by the skeleton.

Dietary fibre and phytate may both impair calcium absorption; it might therefore be supposed that a fibre-rich diet will result in more osteoporosis. However, this is not the case in vegetarians who tend to have less osteoporosis than meat eaters. This may be because the absence of meat in the vegetarian diet causes an alkaline urine, which does not remove calcium.

Fluoride increases the density of the bone; excess fluoride can cause calcification of non-bony tissues. Less osteoporosis is reported in areas where the drinking water contains fluoride ions. Fluoride supplementation has been used with some success in treating patients with established osteoporosis.

A high phosphate consumption is known to reduce calcium absorption and may also increase urinary calcium excretion. The high intake of phosphates in soft drinks may result in lower calcium levels in the bone; these drinks should be avoided by the middle aged, as they may accelerate bone loss. They should not be replaced by alcohol; large amounts are also reported to increase bone loss.

Vitamin D, because of its central role in calcium metabolism, is believed to be involved in the development of osteoporosis. However, the exact picture is not clear, as lack of vitamin D alone can also produce abnormal bone structure – osteomalacia. It seems reasonable to assume that sufficient vitamin D should be provided to facilitate calcium uptake into bones.

(2) *Exercise.* Activity is essential for bone health. Confinement to bed or immobilization leads to bone loss at any age; conversely, activity and movement result in increased bone deposition. Thus physical activity in young adulthood can result in greater bone mass. If this is maintained it will minimize the development of clinical osteoporosis and also help in the maintenance of normal body weight.

(3) *Calcium supplements.* Some studies have shown that calcium intakes between 1000 and 1500 mg are of benefit in preventing calcium loss in middle age. However, other studies have not shown any benefit. Addition of fluoride, vitamin D and oestrogens to the calcium therapy has produced greater benefit. It thus seems that a high calcium intake alone is probably insufficient to maintain bone density in middle age.

In summary, it is probably best to aim for as high a bone mass as possible at the start of the middle years while bone deposition is still possible. This is achieved by a suitable dietary intake and exercise. Exercise commenced in middle age can be of benefit: middle-aged marathon runners have been shown to have 11% more calcium than sedentary contemporaries.

Cardiovascular disease

Deaths attributable to cardiovascular disease account for more than half of the total deaths in many western countries. These include failure of the blood supply to the heart muscle, which causes a heart attack. Inadequate blood supply to a region of the brain results in a stroke. Two separate processes are involved in the development of a heart attack or stroke. The first is the narrowing of arteries by the deposition of a variety of substances over many years; this is known as atherosclerosis. Most commonly affected arteries are those in the brain and heart muscle, and the main leg arteries. The second process is the formation of a blood clot (thrombus) or a haemorrhage. This is likely to be a sudden event, which probably precipitates the actual heart attack or stroke.

Prevention in early or middle life is an important public health measure. The risk factors are described in Chapter 17. For cardiovascular disease, these are both endogenous (i.e. they are part of the individual's biological identity) and exogenous (or environmentally determined and, as such, susceptible to modification). It is the latter group that is focussed on in prevention programmes.

Smoking, hypertension and blood lipid levels are the three major risk factors that have been identified in atherosclerosis.

Smoking is damaging to health in many ways, and stopping smoking is an important health measure. Discussion of this issue is outside the scope of this book.

Hypertension is a common finding in middle age. Healthy young adults have a systolic blood pressure of about 120 mmHg and a diastolic blood pressure of about 80 mmHg; their blood pressure is then expressed as 120/80. In the West, blood pressure rises with age in most people and may reach 160/90 by the age of 60. A diagnosis of hypertension is made when the diastolic blood pressure is greater than

90 mmHg in a younger person, or over 100 mmHg in one over 65 years. High blood pressure is a major contributor to heart attacks and particularly to strokes.

Several factors contribute to hypertension:

(1) There is a hereditary tendency to raised blood pressure; persons with a family history of hypertension require special attention.

(2) There is a close link with overweight. Not every obese person has hypertension, nor is every hypertensive overweight (although 60% are reported to be). However, some overweight hypertensive individuals can reduce their blood pressure by losing weight.

The importance of maintaining normal weight is again apparent. In addition, obesity acquired between the ages of 20 and 40 carries most danger of cardiovascular disease.

(3) Dietary factors.

(a) Salt. There is epidemiological evidence suggesting that chronic high salt (sodium) intakes are associated with hypertension (see Chapter 7). Present evidence suggests that between 9 and 20% of the western population exhibits a genetic sensitivity to salt. In these, a reduction of salt intake would be of benefit in preventing hypertension. In the absence of a screening programme, NACNE recommend an overall salt reduction for the whole population.

(b) Potassium. Low rates of hypertension have also been associated with high potassium intakes. However, use of potassium supplements to lower blood pressure has not shown significant results. Fruit and vegetables are rich sources of potassium, and an increase in their consumption, perhaps in place of processed, salt-rich foods, might be of benefit.

(c) Other factors. Several studies have indicated that increased dietary calcium intakes, and a raised polyunsaturated/saturated fat ratio (of 0.8 to 1.0) with a lower total fat intake, may reduce blood pressure.

There are no firm conclusions to be made in the present state of knowledge about the prevention of hypertension. It would, however, seem desirable to follow healthy eating recommendations with regard to a reduction in processed foods, increased intakes of fruit and vegetables and an adequate level of calcium preferably from low-fat dairy products. Weight control and a general move towards less saturated fat would also be recommended.

Arthritis

There are two main forms of arthritis which affect people in the West: rheumatoid arthritis and osteoarthritis. Both result in disablement, which may subsequently reduce the ability to obtain an adequate dietary intake.

Osteoarthritis is an exaggeration of normal aging in the joints; it tends to affect middle-aged women in a generalized form, particularly affecting the fingers and spine. In more elderly people of both sexes one or two larger joints are more likely to be involved. These may include weight-bearing joints, or those subjected to excessive strain. This strain is increased in overweight; thus weight control by maintenance of activity is essential as a preventive measure. Once the disease process is established, activity may be severely restricted, exacerbating weight gain.

Rheumatoid arthritis is believed to be an autoimmune disorder, in which membranes within the joints become thickened and inflamed resulting in considerable pain. Sufferers may experience weight loss and anaemia. A well-balanced, nutrient-dense diet is important in the management of patients. It is unlikely that dietary prevention measures are relevant. Rheumatoid arthritis is discussed further in Chapter 15.

Cancer

As with most diseases, the incidence of cancer increases with age. It is estimated that up to 80% of cancers in humans are environmentally determined (including dietary influence), and thus are potentially preventable.

The links between diet and cancer are reviewed in Chapter 17. It is relevant to note here that appropriate dietary change for the prevention of cancer may be particularly important in the middle years. This is because many cancers are believed to have a latency period extending to many years, between the first initiation and transformation of the cells into cancer cells, and the ultimate rapid proliferation of the cancer. If the diet is healthy and not conducive to the initiation or proliferation, then the tumour will not grow. Dietary guidelines for the prevention of cancer are summarized in Table 17.6 on page 216.

Summary

Some of the specific nutritional problems that may affect people in their middle years have been explored. It is not intended to give the impression that these problems are exclusive to middle age, nor that dietary change should only occur at this time. However, the middle years are a time of change in an individual's life; there may for the first time be an increased awareness of the risk of disease, with the possibility of an associated motivation to change.

The dietary modifications proposed are not new; they merely expand on the principles of healthy eating described earlier. Special areas of need, including weight control, exercise and the need for calcium, are highlighted.

The elderly

In this discussion the term 'elderly' is used to refer to men and women of pensionable age. In the UK this generally means 65 years or over for men and over 60 years for women. The upper end of the age spectrum for this group is not defined – in the UK there are over 1000 men and women aged 100 years or more (the majority are women). In the 1981 census in the UK, 17.7% of the population were of pensionable age; this amounted to 10.3 million people. The total numbers of elderly persons are increasing in most western countries. In the UK, the major increase in the next 20 years is envisaged in the over-75 age group, and more particularly in the over-85 group. These are the most vulnerable sectors of the retired population, and so it is likely that nutritional problems will increase.

In making general statements about the vulnerability of the elderly population, it is important to remember that there is considerable variation between individuals, as at any age.

Preparation for retirement and a healthy old age should begin earlier in life. It involves the acquisition of healthy eating habits, as described in the section on middle age. Moreover, there should be a healthy life style, involving both physical and mental stimulation. Good nutrition is an important adjunct to both of these. Several studies confirm that health and good nutrition coexist in the elderly; when one begins to deteriorate, often so does the other.

Why are some of the elderly at risk?

Several factors may interact, increasing the likelihood of a nutritional deficiency.

(1) *Inadequate intake.* There are many contributory factors influencing a poor food intake. They can be broadly classified as in Table 13.5.

(a) Physical/medical factors. Aging is often associated with reduced mobility, from rheumatic disease, arthritis, or as a consequence of a stroke, resulting in partial paralysis. It may be sufficiently severe to make the person housebound, or even bedfast. Preparation and eating of food may also be problematical.

Dentition and the state of the mouth also play an important part in food intake. It is reported that some 60% of men and women over the age of 70 have none of their own teeth; a further proportion have partial dentition. Both groups rely on dentures to replace the absent teeth. The selection of foods may be affected, with soft, nutrient-dilute foods eaten and hard foods avoided.

Appetite may be reduced by coexisting disease, or by its treatment. For example, diseases of the gastrointestinal tract, associated with nausea or vomiting, will severely limit appetite. In addition, various drugs used in treatment have a depressing effect on appetite.

Mental illness and depression are also likely to affect the appetite. There may be a complete disregard for eating, with a loss of time sense, so that mealtimes are ignored.

(b) Social factors. Availability of money for the purchase of food is perhaps the most important factor affecting food intake in many elderly people. The retired usually have a fixed income. They may spend in excess of 30% of their income on food: this compares with an average figure in the UK of about 20%.

Lack of education, both about organizing a limited budget and about nutrition, increases vulnerability for some. As in every age group, there will be elderly people who can make a limited budget stretch to cope with expenses, and others who are less good at this. The degree to which present-day nutritional ideas have been recognized and adopted by the elderly is likely to depend on their own level of education and open-mindedness.

Table 13.5 Factors contributing to a poor food intake in the elderly.

Physical/medical factors	Social factors	Psychological factors
Mobility	Money available	Depression
Selection of foods bought	Food storage/preparation facilities	Bereavement
Food preparation	Education/knowledge of nutrition	Mental illness
Dentition	Social isolation	Alcoholism
Appetite		
disease		
drugs		

The elderly, more than any other age group, may become socially isolated. Retirement removes the social contact provided by employment. In addition, there is a tradition of moving away to a 'retirement home', perhaps in a new area. This breaking of social ties may result in a period of friendlessness. As people age, increasing numbers of their friends and relatives die. The splitting of the nuclear family increases the isolation. Most vulnerable to isolation are the housebound.

Several studies have shown that food intake was less and nutritional status poorer among those living alone and experiencing isolation. In particular, the widowed and men were more severely affected than the life-long single and women. Conversely, where an effort was made to share food and eat in company, the food intake was better.

(c) Psychological factors. Depression, often caused by bereavement, is probably one of the major causes of inadequate food intake in an otherwise healthy person. This may persist for many years, leading to malnutrition. Altered mental function, with memory loss and unusual behaviour, may also occur and is likely to result in erratic eating. Severely demented patients are cared for in hospitals and long-stay institutions, where food is provided. However, some of the nutritional problems of institutionalization may then become apparent.

Some elderly people may cope with bereavement or isolation by consuming large amounts of alcohol. The problems associated with alcoholism may be aggravated by, and in turn aggravate, the problems of aging.

(2) *Less efficient digestion/absorption*. Relatively little is known about the effects of aging on the functioning of the digestive tract. There is believed to be a reduced secretion of hydrochloric acid in the stomach, which may limit the efficiency of gastric digestion, particularly with reference to iron. Reduced enzyme production may have an effect on pancreatic juice in particular. There may also be minor malabsorption syndromes, associated with a decrease in the intestinal mucosal surface and broader, shorter villi. Absorption may also be reduced as a result of chronic laxative use. The extent of these changes in a normal elderly person is however unknown.

(3) *Altered needs*. Many bodily functions become less efficient with aging. For example, there is evidence that nutrient uptake by cells can decrease with age. Thus an apparently adequate intake for a younger person may not produce the same nutrient level in the cells in an elderly person. By the same token, supplementation with nutrients may produce disappointing results.

It is well recognized that energy needs decrease with aging, due to the reduction in basal metabolic rate and activity. However, it has been suggested that elderly subjects need more protein than younger adults to maintain protein balance.

The presence of disease, and its treatment by drugs, may also affect nutritional needs. The effects may be magnified by drug interactions. Further problems may arise in a confused patient who fails to take drugs at prescribed times.

Up to 60% of drugs taken by the elderly are obtained without prescription, from the pharmacy. One of the commonest is aspirin, which interferes with the absorption of vitamin C and may cause bleeding along the gut. It may thus cause a vitamin C deficiency or an anaemia. Laxatives, also frequently obtained without prescription, can deplete the body of potassium, causing depression and abnormal heart function.

Does nutritional deficiency occur in the elderly?

A study of elderly people in the UK by the DHSS in 1979 identified 7.1% who were clinically malnourished, with deficiencies of vitamins C and D, and anaemias of multiple aetiology, particularly including folate. In all of the cases, medical or social factors had contributed to the deficiency. The most important medical factors were chronic bronchitis, emphysema, depression and dentition; of the social factors, low socio-economic status, having no regular cooked meals and bereavement were the most important. In this survey, the housebound and those over 80 were found to be at greater risk than the rest of the group.

Several studies have indicated that vitamin C intakes may be sufficiently low to cause scurvy in 0.2 to 0.8% of the elderly; subclinical scurvy causing less well-defined symptoms may be even more widespread. Those at greatest risk are men living alone, and elderly persons in long-stay institutions.

Vitamin D deficiency resulting in osteomalacia may occur in 2 to 5% of the elderly in poor health (admitted to hospital), and in 0.5% of the general elderly population. The most important contribution to vitamin D status is made by sunlight; two weeks' holiday in the summer, with plenty of time spent out of doors, is the most effective way of achieving good vitamin D status. Fatty fish eaten weekly can make a useful but less marked contribution. Exposure to sunlight at a window can make a difference to vitamin D status; the housebound remain the most at risk.

Folic acid deficiency results in megaloblastic anaemia in 1 to 2% of those over 70 years old. Those who are most likely to be at risk are those suffering also from chronic illness, dementia and alcoholism. Other nutritional deficits may also exist in all of these conditions. Anaemia was identified in about 7% of the sample of elderly people in DHSS surveys, although low iron intakes did not appear to be responsible. In many cases the anaemia was of multiple aetiology. Defects in metabolism of the iron, cell synthesis, or chronic, small blood losses, may all contribute to the anaemia.

Low potassium intake has been shown to exist among a group of elderly recipients of 'meals on wheels' in the UK. An independent assessment identified a number of depressed subjects as having a lower mean potassium intake than those who were not depressed. Once depression has resulted from a low potassium intake, this may in turn lead to a further decline in appetite and interest in food.

Probably the most common nutritional disorder among the elderly in western society is obesity. As at·any other age, this is multifactorial in origin and is detrimental to health. If the overweight is of very longstanding, the likelihood of successful, significant weight loss in an elderly person is small. Nonetheless, in cases of diabetes, hypertension and arthritis, weight loss is desirable and should be actively encouraged.

What can be done for the elderly?

In the ideal situation, no elderly person would become nutritionally 'at risk'. This is unlikely ever to be the case, as many of the causative factors are associated with disease and general ill health, as well as the physiological process of aging.

It is necessary to identify those at risk as rapidly and efficiently as possible, before they enter a spiral of deficiency and inadequate intake, leading to further deficiency. Ten major risk factors have been identified (Table 13.6). The presence

Table 13.6 Major risk factors indicating vulnerability in an elderly person.

The presence of several of the following
suggests possible nutritional problems:

Depression/loneliness
Fewer than 8 protein-containing meals per week
Long periods without food
Little milk drunk
High level of food wastage
Disease or disability
Low income
Inability to shop
Sudden weight change
Fruit and vegetables seldom included in the diet.

of several of these factors points to increased nutritional vulnerability and the need
for intervention.

The support services available in the UK include the provision of luncheon
clubs and day centres for those who are reasonably mobile, and 'meals on wheels'
and home helps for those elderly who cannot get out, or are incapable of fully
looking after themselves. These provide some social contact, as well as helping the
nutritional status. Luncheon clubs and day centres provide a midday meal and
generally some form of social activity, which may also have a therapeutic role.
Most importantly, they provide social contact, thus helping the mental attitude.
At the same time, a balanced meal contributes to a reasonable nutrient intake.

The elderly in institutions

Of the elderly in the UK, 5% are cared for in institutions. These are the most
vulnerable subgroup: it is because they are ill, infirm and incapable of caring for
themselves that they are in the hospitals and homes for the elderly. Disease is more
likely to be present in this group, with associated altered needs. The diet provided
may be nutritionally incomplete, particularly with respect to vitamins C and D,
although other nutrients have also been shown to be low. There may be problems
with eating, swallowing and appetite. Many disease processes may make nutritional adequacy difficult to achieve, or measure. However, every effort should be
made to ensure that the elderly in institutions are properly fed.

Although some of the elderly population encounter nutritional problems, it
should be remembered that the great majority live a reasonably healthy life and
succeed in caring adequately for themselves. A positive outlook and a continued
interest in life are important prerequisites. When interest in food wanes and food
intake declines, a decline in health will surely follow.

14

Nutrition and Other Special Groups

There are certain situations in the lives of individuals that put them nutritionally 'at risk'. This may be as a result of a reduced or altered food intake, poorer absorption of nutrients, increased needs for nutrients, or because greater amounts of nutrients are being lost from the body.

Pregnant women

During pregnancy a woman's diet has to provide sufficient nutrients both for the maintenance of her own body and the foetus in her womb. During the nine months of pregnancy, the mother's weight increases by an average of 12.5 kg. This comprises:

Foetus	3.5 kg
Increased maternal tissue (including uterus, breasts, blood volume)	5.0 kg
Stored fat	4.0 kg
	12.5 kg

The successful outcome of a pregnancy, in terms of a healthy, well-developed, normal weight baby and a healthy mother, is largely dependent on the mother's nutrition during the pregnancy.

Several features of the pre-pregnancy diet may also affect the chances of conception or the success of the pregnancy. Vitamin D deficiency in adolescence may have resulted in rickets with pelvic malformations, making normal delivery impossible.

If the usual eating pattern is unbalanced or generally unhealthy, the woman's body may not be well prepared (in terms of nutrient reserves) for the added needs of pregnancy. In this case, it would be advantageous to improve the general food intake pattern before becoming pregnant. It would also provide a sound foundation for family eating in years to come.

Very underweight women are often infertile. As weight increases towards normal, fertility usually returns. It has been suggested that a critical body fat content of 12 kg is necessary before a normal pregnancy can be sustained. Thus girls and women who are restricting their food intakes to lose weight may be at increased risk here.

At the other end of the weight spectrum, the very overweight woman may also have difficulty in conceiving. If she does, then there are greater risks and complications associated with pregnancy, both for the mother and her baby.

A healthy diet ensures adequate nutritional status at conception. It may be especially important in women who have been taking the contraceptive pill and now want to become pregnant. The 'pill' leads to some abnormal levels of vitamins in the body, by affecting their absorption and metabolism, and it is recommended that at least three months is allowed after stopping the 'pill' prior to conception, to allow these levels to return to normal.

Nutrition during pregnancy

This would appear to be the most important time for good nutrition to be practised. The mother's body must provide all the needs of a growing foetus.

The needs of the foetus are not uniform throughout the pregnancy; they are relatively small during the first six months and increase in the last three months. This is in parallel with its size, which increases rapidly during the last three months of the pregnancy.

To cope with this pattern of demand by the foetus, the mother's body undergoes various physiological adaptations. These increase her own efficiency of metabolism, so that a greater use is made of the nutrients available to her. These include:

(1) A fall in her basal metabolic rate in early pregnancy, allowing energy to be saved for later use by the foetus.

(2) More efficient protein metabolism in the first part of pregnancy, so that more can be incorporated into the tissues and then released, for use by the foetus in the second part of pregnancy.

(3) Hormonal levels increase to help the mobilization of calcium from the bones, to supplement that available from the diet.

(4) Iron is taken from the stores in the bone marrow to provide for the increase in red blood cell numbers which occurs around the middle part of pregnancy.

(5) The muscular activity of the intestines slows down, so that food spends a longer time being digested and absorbed, thus allowing for a more efficient usage.

This slowed activity of the intestines may cause heartburn and constipation. Heartburn arises because the muscles at the top of the stomach are more relaxed, which allows reflux of the acid stomach contents into the lower part of the oesophagus, causing pain.

Constipation occurs because of the greater absorption of nutrients and water from the intestines. Increasing both the fluid and the dietary fibre intakes can help to relieve this problem.

In these ways, the high nutrient needs of late pregnancy are spread over a longer period of time.

Appetite

The mother's appetite is a good guide to her overall needs for energy.

In the first three months of pregnancy many women (up to 70%) suffer from nausea and vomiting. Although this is commonly termed 'morning sickness' it can actually occur at any time of day or night – and in some women occurs continuously. It may range from a mild nausea to quite severe, frequent vomiting. Very frequent meals or snacks are recommended even if the woman has little appetite for them. Overall food intake may be quite low at this time, which matches the nutritional needs.

During the middle part of pregnancy appetite is generally good, so that food intake is at or a little above normal non-pregnant levels. This ensures an adequate provision of energy and nutrients, to form a reserve for the greater needs of the last three months.

In the last three months the needs of the foetus are high and the mother's appetite may increase, to take in perhaps an extra 1200 kJ per day. She is however limited in her capacity for food, because of pressure of the enlarged womb on her stomach.

What should pregnant women eat?

From what has already been said, it should be obvious that a pregnant woman does *not* need to 'eat for two'.

There is no single, special diet for pregnancy: a healthy, well-balanced diet containing a complete range of nutrients is sufficient. The actual amounts of food need be no higher than usual in the first three months, but should increase slightly in the second and slightly more in the last three-month period.

Although all nutrients are provided by a mixed diet, there are three to which particular attention should be paid. These are calcium, and vitamins C and D, whose recommended levels (according to *Report 15*) are increased proportionately more than those of energy and the other nutrients. Taking extra milk or dairy products will provide additional calcium and vitamin D; increased fruit and vegetable intake will provide extra vitamin C in the diet.

The inclusion of fruits and vegetables in greater amounts will also improve the intake of folate and dietary fibre. It has been reported that folate intakes are low in the UK, although analysis techniques are known to be inaccurate; pregnancy is an especially vulnerable time for low folate status. Thus a higher intake could be advantageous. Up to 25% of women in the UK are reported to have insufficient folate in late pregnancy, with associated changes in their red blood cells. In many developing countries folate deficiency is a major problem in pregnancy, and supplementation is very desirable. Folate-deficient mothers are likely to deliver premature, low-birthweight infants.

Dietary fibre is an important constituent of the diet at all times, but especially useful in pregnancy where there is a tendency to constipation.

Certain individual women will have particular needs for dietary supplements, for example of energy, protein, iron, folate and vitamin D. These are exceptional conditions and are not considered further here.

When alcohol is drunk regularly, at a level of more than 10 drinks per week, it can cause some developmental damage to the baby (1 drink = half a pint of beer, a single spirit measure or one glass of wine, sherry, etc.). The exact amount of alcohol at which this can occur is unknown and probably varies between different women. It is, however, clear that women who drink heavily run a great risk of having a baby which suffers from 'foetal alcohol syndrome', with a whole array of malformations. The safest advice is to avoid alcohol in pregnancy, or at least to limit drinking to fewer than 8 drinks per week. 'Binge' drinking, with irregular intakes of alcohol, can be equally dangerous.

The nursing or lactating mother

Breast feeding a newborn infant is the natural sequel to pregnancy. The process of lactation (or milk production) does not occur in isolation; the mother's breasts become prepared for lactation during pregnancy.

In addition the mother's body has a store of some 4 kg of fat, which is available for use as an energy source during lactation.

The process of lactation

There are two stages involved in this process:

(1) *Milk production or secretion.* Milk is made by the mammary glands in the breasts, by appropriate transfer of specific nutrients from the blood into the gland.

(2) *Milk ejection or let-down.* The milk once formed is not immediately released from the breasts. The normal release of milk occurs when the baby suckles at the breast and initiates a reflex in the mother. It is believed that the stimulus of suckling by the baby is an essential trigger for the ejection or let-down reflex. This reflex can be influenced by the mother's mental state. If she is apprehensive or unhappy at the prospect of breast feeding, this can inhibit the let-down reflex and make the process of feeding unsuccessful.

Diet in lactation

As with pregnancy, there is no special diet for lactation. It must be remembered, however, that the food eaten by the mother in the first 4 to 6 months of breast feeding (before the baby starts taking any food other than milk), has to meet her own needs and all the needs of the baby, which are considerably greater than its needs while in the womb.

Energy. The average daily volume of milk produced varies from mother to mother. Data from around the world suggest a figure of 850 ml, once lactation is fully established (at about 2 to 3 months). It has been calculated that 3.1 MJ of energy are used each day in milk production.

Some of this energy can be met from the 4 kg of fat stored during pregnancy. It is thought to be used up gradually at about 900 kJ per day, partially supplying the energy needs of lactation for six months. The remaining 2.2 MJ must be supplied from the diet.

An incidental benefit is that the additional body weight gained during pregnancy will be lost without the need for a weight-reducing diet.

Often a breast-feeding mother experiences an increased appetite, which ensures that additional food is eaten. In many communities in the world, however, food supply may normally be inadequate to meet recommended levels. The effects of this apparent shortfall of energy for the lactation process have been studied in various communities. It seems that lactation can occur satisfactorily even in these apparently adverse circumstances. However, the nutritional content of the milk probably starts to fall from the third or fourth month of lactation. This does not happen in an adequately nourished woman.

Protein. The protein in milk supplies the necessary amino acids for the growth of the baby. This protein must eventually derive from maternal protein – in turn supplied by the mother's diet. The calculated additional protein required (17.5 g) can be met from the increased food intake eaten to supply the extra energy. In other words, as long as the extra energy is supplied by a normal, mixed diet (and not a concentrated source of energy such as sugar), then this will automatically provide the increment of protein. On a poor diet, where the total food supply is inadequate, there may be no additional protein, but protein levels in the milk are maintained for several months, even under these circumstances.

Calcium and vitamin D. The amount of calcium secreted each day in milk is 300 mg. To meet this demand an intake of 1200 mg is recommended – the same as for the last three months of pregnancy. It can readily be met from additional milk or dairy products in the diet. In the UK the average calcium intake already approaches 1000 mg in the adult population, so no great change needs to be made to the average diet. If calcium intakes are inadequate the milk content of this mineral will be maintained at the expense of the mother's skeleton.

As an essential aid to the increased turnover of calcium, the body also requires sufficient vitamin D. This facilitates calcium absorption from the diet and helps to maintain serum calcium levels. The vitamin may be obtained by synthesis in the skin under the influence of ultraviolet light. When no skin synthesis can occur, dietary sources are important; this is particularly the case in the winter months in northern latitudes (e.g. in the UK).

Women whose vitamin D status is borderline may need to receive a supplement, to ensure normal calcium metabolism.

Vitamin A. Milk contains approximately 450 μg of vitamin A in the average volume secreted daily. The mother's dietary intake of vitamin A should be increased to enable her to supply this amount of the vitamin.

General requirements. If the mother satisfies her need for additional energy, then the increased needs for all the other nutrients should be met, assuming that the extra food eaten is well balanced. Nutrients that might warrant particular attention are calcium and vitamin D; foods containing these should be present regularly in the diet.

If it is not possible to increase food intake, then the nutritional quality of the milk may suffer. The water-soluble vitamins (B complex and C) will be present in smaller amounts, reflecting poorer maternal status. The other constituents, namely fats, lactose, protein and fat-soluble vitamins, may be maintained at an adequate level for 3 to 4 months, but will then decline. The weight gain of the baby may slow down or stop at this point and alternative sources of food will be needed for the baby.

Early stopping of breast feeding increases the likelihood of another conception. The mother may then embark on another pregnancy and lactation, with no opportunity to restore her own nutritional reserves.

Thus good nutrition during lactation contributes not only to the immediate welfare of the baby, but also to the longer-term well-being of the mother and her family.

Immigrants

Many people around the world, for a variety of political or economic reasons, move to and settle in a country that is not their own. In doing so they become immigrants to that country.

If the culture of the host country is similar to that of the immigrant's own mother country, settlement is relatively easy. If there are many cultural, religious and language differences, the immigrant may experience problems of acceptance and acceptability in the host community.

Food habits are an important cultural aspect and their significance is explored in Chapter 12. Because many immigrants keep to their traditional food habits in the host country, they may encounter some nutritional problems. These are likely to be the result of the coexistence of a number of factors, only some of which are nutritional, which lead to deficiencies in the diet.

These problems are described with reference to the main groups of immigrants to the United Kingdom: Europeans (including those of Eastern European and Mediterranean origins), Asians from the Indian subcontinent, people of Afro-Caribbean origin, Chinese and (most recently) a relatively small number of Vietnamese.

The Europeans, together with the small groups of immigrants from most other parts of the globe, have not been found to experience nutritional difficulties or possible deficiencies in Britain.

Features common to most immigrant groups

Most new immigrants share the common feature of belonging to a socially disadvantaged sector of society.

This may be reflected in various aspects of life, including low income, unemployment, poor housing, poorer educational opportunity, and less acess to health care. All of these are likely to have a bearing on nutrition. Where the traditional diet is maintained, the higher cost of imported foods may limit the amount of food eaten.

The traditional diet may be modified by the substitution of some British foods, to replace unavailable traditional items. Unfortunately, the British foods chosen are often those of poorest nutritional quality, such as the highly refined and processed items, which are not nutritionally comparable to the traditional items they are replacing. In this way, a well-balanced traditional diet, by attempting to become integrated into the British diet, becomes nutritionally inferior. It is important that where some adaptation to the British diet occurs, the foods chosen should be nutritionally adequate.

For the children of some of the immigrant groups, school meals pose a major dilemma. If they have been brought up eating only a traditional diet, foods presented in school may be completely unfamiliar, both in content and style of presentation. With time, peer pressure may encourage these children to sample some British foods. If they enjoy them, they may eventually request them at home.

In many areas, the school meals service provides menus which comply with the dietary laws of some ethnic groups. In this case the food education can work in two directions – the children of the host country have the opportunity to broaden their eating experience with food typical of other lands, while the immigrant children may taste their traditional foods made from local ingredients.

Asian immigrants

Much attention has been focussed on the Asian immigrants from Bangladesh, India or Pakistan. In addition, a smaller number of Asian immigrants came to

Britain from African countries such as Uganda and Kenya.

Religion is an important aspect of life for these groups and most are followers of one of the three major religions found in Asia: Hinduism, Islam or Sikhism. These have specific dietary laws which have possible nutritional implications.

Hinduism. This is an ancient religion, one of whose main precepts is the sanctity of life and the transmigration of the soul. Associated with this is a prohibition on the taking of life, including that of an animal for food. Thus Hindus are vegetarians, eating only plant foods, and any animal foods which do not involve killing – for example dairy products. Eggs may be avoided by some Hindus, particularly women, as they are seen as a potential source of life. The cow is deemed sacred; its products are prized in the diet. Orthodox Hindus will adhere strictly to dietary laws, but some who are less orthodox may eat some meat, although usually not beef or pork (the pig is considered unclean).

Fasting, which means either total abstinence from food or alternatively the eating of 'pure' foods – fruit, yoghurt, nuts and potatoes – may be a regular occurrence.

Islam. Followers of Islam are Muslims. The religious teachings in the Koran cover most aspects of life, including dietary laws, as well as rules on fasting.

Muslims are permitted to eat the flesh of ruminant animals, (this excludes pork), poultry and fish (excluding shellfish). The animals must be ritually slaughtered; the meat is then described as 'halal'. There are a number of approved 'halal' butchers in the UK. Milk and dairy products are not a major part of the Muslim diet in the UK; they are eaten increasingly as the diet becomes anglicized. Although meat is allowed in the Muslim diet, the amount actually eaten may not be very great, particularly by women.

Asian meals may consist largely of the staple (a rice or wheat dish), together with one or several side dishes which provide the garnish (or flavour) part of the meal.

All Muslims over the age of responsibility (early adolescence) are required to fast daily, from sunrise to sunset, for a four-week period each year; this is known as Ramadan. The actual number of hours of fasting each day in Britain varies with the time of year when Ramadan actually falls. When it occurs in the summer there may be up to sixteen hours of fasting each day; in the winter, the fast may only last for eight hours.

Sikhism. This religion developed comparatively recently (in the sixteenth century) and incorporates some features of both Hinduism and Islam. Dietary restrictions are less than in either of these religions; eggs or meat are not prohibited, but some Sikhs believe in the transmigration of the soul and therefore may be vegetarian.

Very few eat beef, and pork is considered unclean, as with the other two religions described here. Animals for meat must be killed in a prescribed manner, by a single blow to the head; the meat thus produced is known as 'khatka' meat.

General features. In all three of these religious groups, Asian women tend to have a more marked domestic role than in the indigenous population. Integration with the British community may thus be slow. Where the women do go out, to work or mix with the local community, traditional cultural practices are most likely to change.

Afro-Caribbean immigrants

Immigrants to Britain from the West Indies are predominantly of African descent, whose cultural background has been influenced by both life in the West Indies and subsequent migration to Britain. Several ethnic subcultures have been identified among these immigrants. In general the traditional West Indian food habits still adhered to by a large proportion of this population pose few nutritional problems.

The diet is largely based on cereals, such as corn, rice and wheat, and starchy vegetables. These are served in the form of spicy stews or soups, containing many different vegetables. Many of the traditional foods such as mangoes, breadfruit, cassava, green bananas, plantains and yams are available in West Indian neighbourhoods, indicating that they remain an important part of the West Indian diet.

Rastafarians are members of the West Indian community who aspire to return to Ethiopia, which is seen as the African homeland. There is a strong adherence to the Bible and a belief that Haile Selassie, the last Emperor of Ethiopia, was the Messiah. Many of the dietary laws are based on a strict interpretation of the Bible. The diet is strictly vegetarian, containing no meat or animal products. It is based predominantly on fruit, vegetables and cereals. However, because pulses are not a major item in the West Indian diet, the vegetables eaten tend to be starchy roots and leafy vegetables, both groups which contain little protein. There is also a lack of vitamin B_{12} in such a diet. In other ways the diet may be considered healthy: 'convenience', processed foods are banned, and alcohol is not permitted.

As with all dietary laws, the degree of adherence to the diet may vary. However, as Rastafarianism is perceived as conferring an identity to the individual, there is considerable motivation to keep the dietary laws. Nutritional deficiencies have been reported among Rastafarians both in Britain and in other countries, including the West Indies. These are considered further in the deficiencies section below.

Chinese immigrants

The Chinese have a food culture very different from the indigenous population, but despite long periods of settlement in Britain, it has remained largely unchanged.

Although some British foods are included in the diet, usually being requested by the children, these form only a small part of the daily intake. The diet includes rice as a staple and meat, fish, fruit and vegetables prepared in many diverse ways.

Food is seen by the Chinese as providing not just nutrients but contributing to the overall balance of the body. This is described in terms of hot and cold properties (*yin* and *yang*). Foods are ascribed such properties according to the effects they are believed to have on the body (not on the actual temperature of the food). In addition, particular stages of life, and conditions such as pregnancy or illness, all alter the body's balance. The food eaten is carefully selected in order to restore harmony to the body. For example, if children eat a school meal which is considered 'hot', they will be given a 'cooling' food on their return home to restore balance. Thus, rather than avoiding British foods, the Chinese simply accommodate them and adjust the other foods eaten accordingly.

There are no reports in the literature of nutritional problems associated with the Chinese diet in Britain.

Vietnamese immigrants

A relatively small number (16 000) of Vietnamese immigrants came to Britain in the late 1970s, having left Vietnam mostly for political reasons. A considerable amount of attention was focussed on this group on their arrival; many aspects of their life were examined, including food practices.

The majority of Vietnamese who have settled in Britain are ethnic Chinese and share many dietary practices with the Chinese as described above. The diet is rice-based, with rice forming the main constituent of each meal. It is accompanied by a number of side dishes, which will contain meat or fish and vegetables. The food is generally selected for its freshness and is lightly cooked by stir-frying or steaming. Sauces and soups form an important addition to the meal and contribute valuable nutrients.

Many common foods available in Britain can be readily incorporated into this diet. In some cases, common items like cabbage may be substituted for the more expensive and less commonly found Chinese leaf. However, there are certain British foods that do not readily fit into the Vietnamese diet; these include root vegetables and tinned fruit. Lamb is unknown in the Vietnamese cuisine and so tends not to be eaten. Conversely, offal (not a popular item among the indigenous population) is frequently included.

Despite these differences in food selection, no nutritional problems have yet been identified among the Vietnamese.

Beliefs about 'hot' and 'cold' properties of food exist among the Vietnamese, as already described for the Chinese. The significance and practical application of these is similar.

Nutritional deficiencies in ethnic minority groups

As a result of social, economic and cultural factors certain members of ethnic minority groups living in Britain are at an increased risk of nutritional deficiency.

This is most likely to occur at times of increased need for nutrients: infancy and early childhood, adolescence and pregnancy. All of these are periods of life when growth is occurring, which increases the physiological requirement for specific nutrients. The nutrients that have been reported to be deficient include vitamin D (and possibly calcium), iron, folic acid and B_{12} (all needed for blood production), and occasionally protein.

Vitamin D deficiency

Rickets and osteomalacia are mainly a problem among the Asian community, where they affect all the groups mentioned above, together with older women. The deficiency has also recently been found in Rastafarian children. Many factors have been put forward in explanation of the prevalence of rickets and osteomalacia in this group.

(1) *Skin pigmentation.* As vitamin D is synthesized in the skin on exposure to ultraviolet light, it has been suggested that increased skin pigmentation reduces penetration of the light rays and hence reduces synthesis. However, measurements of vitamin D synthesized on ultraviolet light exposure by dark-skinned and white-skinned subjects found no difference.

(2) *Outdoor exposure*. Several studies of the Asian community in Britain found that Asian women spent relatively less time outside than their indigenous counterparts. In addition, there was a tendency to be well covered, usually in traditional dress. Other studies have found little difference in outdoor exposure, and thus the significance of this factor is unclear.

(3) *Diet*. Foods containing vitamin D may be completely absent from the traditional Asian diet. Measurements of the effects of various levels of vitamin D intake show that both Asian and indigenous groups have levels that are too small to make any appreciable difference to blood vitamin D content. It therefore appears to be unimportant that the typical Asian intake is lower than that of the white population. Supplementation of dietary vitamin D with drops or tablets, to provide at least 5 μg per day, preferably 10 μg per day, is needed to make a significant impact on the blood levels.

Most studies on the causes of vitamin D deficiency have noted that it is most widespread amongst those whose diet is most strictly vegetarian. Diets which contain no meat, eggs or dairy products appear therefore to be most rachitogenic (rickets-causing) among the Asian population.

It has been suggested that the high dietary fibre and phytate content of these diets reduces the availability of calcium and also may bind vitamin D present in the digestive tract, causing it to be lost in the faeces.

A strict vegetarian diet has recently been implicated in vitamin D deficiency among Rastafarian infants in Britain. Initially breast-fed, these infants were weaned on to a cereal and grain weaning food, without adequate supplementation.

It appears that the factors described above may interact to produce the clinical picture of vitamin D deficiency. The remedies, within the limits of present knowledge, seem to be the inclusion of a little animal produce into the diet and/or supplementation with vitamin D.

Anaemia

Anaemia most usually arises from an inadequate intake of iron, folic acid or vitamin B_{12}, or a combination of these.

Among the ethnic minorities in Britain, anaemias have been found among infants, young children and in pregnant women.

Iron deficiency. In infancy it is most commonly the result of prolonged milk feeding, or of weaning on to foods that are predominantly starchy and contain little iron.

This situation has been found among Asian immigrants, Rastafarians and occasionally other West Indians. Sometimes children of other immigrant groups have also developed anaemia due to a lack of understanding of the rôle of weaning foods.

Pregnant women of all cultures are at risk of iron deficiency anaemia, particularly if their body iron stores are low when pregnancy begins.

The existence of low stores is more likely when the diet is vegetarian, or contains little meat. Iron tablets may be routinely prescribed during the antenatal period, but women from the ethnic minority groups are less likely to attend for antenatal care, particularly if there is a language barrier, and may in addition be reluctant to take iron supplements.

Particularly vulnerable are the Hindu Asian women, who are vegetarian, and Rastafarians.

Folic acid deficiency. Folic acid deficiency is a particular problem of pregnant women, as requirements for the vitamin are raised during periods of rapid cell division. Folic acid is readily destroyed by cooking; its content in leafy vegetables also declines on storage. Thus in ethnic minority groups where vegetables are commonly cooked for a long period of time, and also reheated from day to day, folic acid may be destroyed. Finally, in a vegetarian diet there is complete reliance on these sources for folic acid provision, which may thus be insufficient.

Thus the vegetarian Asian and the Rastafarian are again the most vulnerable. Supplementation with folic acid is available in pregnancy, for those who are identified as at risk.

Vitamin B_{12} deficiency has been reported mainly in Rastafarians, and Hindu women in pregnancy.

Vitamin B_{12} is obtained in foods of animal origin and is needed in very small amounts. It is believed that some bacterial contamination of food may provide sufficient vitamin to prevent an overt deficiency. Vitamin B_{12} deficiency has been reported among Rastafarian men in Jamaica who had consumed a strict vegetarian diet for many years.

In Britain, the most likely group to develop vitamin B_{12} deficiency are Hindu women during pregnancy, when the needs are increased but the vegan diet does not provide the vitamin.

Protein deficiency

Protein deficiency has been seen on a few occasions in infants of ethnic minority groups in Britain. In most cases it had been part of a more complex deficiency picture, usually including iron deficiency as well as multiple vitamin deficiencies. In the majority of cases, the deficiencies have been attributable to inappropriate weaning. The child has been fed exclusively on a dilute starchy food, or simply on milk; both of these provide insufficient energy, so any protein they might contain will be used for energy.

Overnutrition

Despite the occurrence of the deficiencies described above, it should be remembered that the ethnic minority groups in Britain may also suffer from the diseases of overnutrition found in this country – obesity, coronary heart disease and cancer.

It is perhaps unfortunate that some of the healthy eating patterns which ethnic minority groups such as the Chinese bring with them become altered – often for the worse – by the host food practices in Britain. As a result the diet becomes unbalanced, and eventually the immigrants develop the same problems as the indigenous population.

Athletics and sport

In recent years there has been an upsurge of interest in physical activity as a part of a healthy life style. This has included organized activities such as exercise groups and classes, a greater number of people participating in sports such as racquet games or swimming, as well as a growing band of runners.

There is good evidence that some physical activity can protect against certain western diseases. A ten-year follow-up of a study of 18 000 British male civil servants showed that those who took vigorous exercise in their leisure time had less than a quarter of the fatal heart attacks seen in the inactive group.

Activity is also beneficial in weight control; it is likely to reduce the amount of body fat, increase the amount of lean tissue and result in an increased rate of metabolism.

Benefits of activity were recognized by the NACNE (1983) and COMA (1984) reports, for the prevention of overweight and protection against heart disease. Neither of these reports recommended any special diet for people engaging in sport and increased physical activity. So the normal, healthy diet as recommended by NACNE is suitable for sportsmen and women, and can be applied to the needs of the amateur taking part in competition at the athletic or sports club level, as well as to the not-so-young businessman concerned about his state of health who decides to start running.

It may seem surprising that the principles of feeding these apparently different individuals are the same, when the sports literature is full of articles about special diets and products which are 'indispensable' to the athlete. Athletes can be very vulnerable and susceptible to a succession of dietary fads and ideas. If they could be persuaded to adopt a sound, healthy diet, it would remove a whole area of worry from the training programme and allow them to concentrate on the physical training aspects.

Energy

The key consideration in any sports performance is the need for additional energy. This is additional to the energy needed for maintaining normal metabolism and everyday activities.

The additional energy requirement is determined by both the intensity of the activity and its duration. Few athletes will require more than 20 MJ/day; it is estimated that marathon runners may have a daily energy need of approximately 14.6 MJ.

Finding the appropriate energy intake level is important: too little energy is likely to reduce performance, too much will cause weight gain.

Carbohydrate stored in the muscles as glycogen is the major determinant of the amount of exercise that can be performed. Muscle glycogen, together with fatty acids brought to the muscles from stored fat, is the fuel used during exercise; the glycogen and fat are used together, but the amount of glycogen limits the duration of exercise. Athletes therefore need to make the glycogen last for as long as possible. A practice called 'carbohydrate loading' which contributes to an increased amount of available glycogen, has been used for a number of years and has gained in popularity recently.

Factors affecting the usage of glycogen

(1) *Intensity of exercise.* The rate of glycogen use is related to the intensity of exercise: the greater the intensity, the more glycogen is used.

(2) *Duration of the exercise.* In general, there is an increase in the amount of fat used and a relative fall in glycogen usage with increasing duration of exercise.
(3) *Training.* This increases the capacity for fat oxidization, thus spreading glycogen usage over a longer period of time.
(4) *The composition of the pre-exercise diet.* Many studies have shown that the fuels used during exercise (i.e. glycogen or fat) and their proportions can be significantly influenced by the diet eaten before the exercise. Studies on exercising subjects showed that whereas on a normal mixed diet, exercise time to exhaustion was approximately 110 minutes, on a high fat/high protein diet this was reduced to less than 60 minutes, and increased to 166 minutes with a high carbohydrate diet (60–70% carbohydrate energy). These variations in the capacity for exercise were associated with parallel changes in the muscle glycogen content.

The practice of 'carbohydrate loading' enables athletes to increase muscle glycogen in preparation for specific events of more than 60 minutes' duration. This involves exercising to exhaustion, and then eating a high-carbohydrate diet for three days. This diet will contain approximately 60% of the energy as carbohydrate, 10 to 15% protein and 25 to 30% fat. It does *not* mean eating a normal, mixed diet and adding extra carbohydrate to this, as excess energy would be eaten. The carbohydrate should preferably be starch rather than sugar, and so the diet usually includes cereals and their products and starchy vegetables.

This regime has been used successfully in distance running, cycling and in team sports such as hockey and football.

Although the carbohydrate loading regime is recommended only for exercise in excess of 60 minutes' duration, those who exercise regularly but for a shorter duration can experience a cumulative depletion of muscle glycogen. Over a number of days, the glycogen store becomes gradually lower, with only a small repletion during the time between exercise. This repletion can be speeded up by a high-carbohydrate diet, so that the glycogen level is kept 'topped up' and does not fall to 'fatigue' levels. A rest day is also recommended every 4 to 5 days, so that muscle glycogen can return to pre-exercise values.

It is reported that during a rest period with no exercise, a high carbohydrate diet can restore pre-exercise levels of muscle glycogen in 46 hours.

If carbohydrate intakes are low, there is a danger of residual fatigue between training sessions which can reduce morale.

Hence for both the serious athlete and the weekend jogger, an adequate carbohydrate intake is necessary; this should represent 55 to 60% of total energy, and is thus in line with NACNE recommendations. It is important to stress that simple carbohydrate such as glucose should not be taken in the immediate pre-exercise period, as it speeds up glycogen use and shortens the time to its depletion, thus reducing the duration of exercise.

Protein

Many athletes believe that to make full use of their muscles in exercise they require a high protein intake. This stems from the idea that muscles are used up in some way by exercise, and therefore should be replenished from an extra protein intake.

Protein makes a very small contribution to energy supply in exercise and is hardly used up at all. However, an exercising muscle does increase in mass over a period of time, so that when a person first starts to take regular exercise, more protein will initially be retained by the body. In the West, protein intakes are normally higher than the minimum requirement of the body. A western athlete is therefore already likely to be ingesting some additional protein. Additional food to supply the extra energy required, will also provide any additional protein needed.

A reasonable target to aim for is a level of 1 to 1.5 g of protein per kg of body weight, to supply between 10% and 15% of total energy. There is no particular advantage in eating animal protein sources; there are very many successful vegetarian athletes.

Vitamin supplements

There is little evidence that vitamin supplements are of any benefit in adequately nourished persons. Studies which have been published showing some improvements in performance made no assessment of the initial dietary intakes of the subjects, and therefore their findings proved little.

There is likely to be no improvement in performance in an athlete whose initial intake is adequate. From the nutritional standpoint, it would be more desirable if the overall diet was improved, rather than 'patching up' a poor diet with vitamin supplements. There is also a possible risk from excessively high intakes of vitamins such as B_6 and C in certain individuals.

Mineral supplements

Sweat contains a number of ions (electrolytes) in water. In decreasing order of magnitude, these include sodium, chloride, potassium, calcium and magnesium. The physiological purpose of sweating is to cool the body: as the water evaporates, it removes heat from the skin and allows the body to maintain a normal temperature.

The amount of sweat produced varies between individuals and is also determined by the rate of working and the environmental temperature.

The water loss causes dehydration, which can be critical if not replaced; water replacement is a top priority after exercise, or during a long period of exercise. The changes in electrolyte levels are far less critical. In most cases, the total amount of electrolytes in the plasma will be automatically replenished from one day's normal food intake. There is therefore no need for electrolyte replacement drinks. A small amount of glucose (2.5 g/dl) and a maximum of 0.5 g salt/dl water will speed up water absorption from the digestive tract and bring about more rapid rehydration.

Conclusion

In summary, the principles of nutrition for exercise and sport are the same as those of a healthy diet for the whole population. The energy needs may be higher, and much of this energy should be provided by carbohydrates rather than fats. This is in line with current healthy eating guidelines. Once the energy needs are satisfied, the other nutrients largely take care of themselves. If a balanced diet is eaten in sufficient quantity, there is no need for special supplements.

Alcoholics and drug users

When people take large amounts of alcohol, or one of the 'street' drugs, they run the risk of compromising their nutritional status (street drugs are those which are obtained from dealers, rather than through normal medical channels, on prescription from a pharmacist; they include cannabis, heroin and cocaine).

Since there are many more people affected by excessive use of alcohol than by drugs, this discussion will concentrate more on the alcohol users; many factors however are common to both.

The term 'alcoholic' is used to mean a person whose health is being damaged by their intake of alcohol.

Both alcohol and drug use can seriously affect food intake.

(1) There is likely to be a reduced appetite or an overall lack of interest in food, as a result of preoccupation with alcohol or the drug. In the case of the alcoholic the appetite may be further reduced by vomiting because of inflammation of the stomach (gastritis), or simply a large intake of drink. Drug addicts without a regular supply may also vomit during withdrawal.

(2) Money is more likely to be spent on alcohol or drugs, than on food.

(3) The opportunity to obtain food may be limited, and food provision is relegated to a position of little importance. For an addict or alcoholic living with their family, some food may be provided and at least a reasonable intake maintained.

Alcohol is an irritant to living tissue. Regular ingestion causes a permanent state of inflammation along the digestive tract, with vomiting and diarrhoea. Consequently the process of digestion becomes inefficient, as gut contents are moved more rapidly along the tract. In addition enzyme secretion is reduced, with the result that less digestion actually takes place.

Further along the tract, inflammation of the absorptive areas of the small intestine reduces their efficiency with consequent loss of nutrients in the faeces.

An alcoholic or drug addict may also become nutritionally deficient because of changes in the body's metabolism as a result of the alcohol or drug. Liver damage is well recognized as a consequence of alcohol abuse; the liver is also the site of activation, metabolism and storage of many of the nutrients in the body. These actions may be seriously affected, with resultant nutritional disturbances. Some nutrients are used specifically in the metabolism and detoxification of alcohol; their turnover is increased. Additionally, alcohol is a diuretic, increasing urine production. Many water-soluble nutrients may be lost in increased amounts in the urine.

Maintaining a reasonable food intake can help maintain a measure of health. Once food intake deteriorates, then ill health is more likely.

Drug addicts in particular are at increased risk of infection. This can further reduce their food intake. In turn, the poor food intake can increase susceptibility to infection, by reducing resistance.

Energy

Alcoholic drinks provide some energy, but this is in the form of 'empty energy'. If they displace other foods from the diet, the drink itself might still supply enough to meet daily needs. This entails drinking a large volume daily; since alcohol supplies 29 MJ/g, then 400 g of alcohol are needed to supply 11.2 MJ. This would come from, approximately, 20 pints of beer or 40 single measures of spirits.

If food is eaten in addition to the alcoholic drink, the alcoholic may become over-weight. Thus overweight or weight loss may be seen in alcoholics; which of these occurs depends on the total energy intake from the alcohol and food.

The oxidation of alcohol by the liver supplies this organ with energy. Consequently this affects its handling of other sources of energy.

A drug addict is likely to have a low supply of energy and therefore lose weight, unless food intake is being maintained.

Fats

In normal metabolism, fat digestion products brought to the liver are metabolized and subsequently distributed to the adipose tissue around the body. In alcoholics the removal of fat from the liver becomes inefficient, so that fat accumulates here, leading to the formation of a fatty liver. There are also raised levels of circulating lipids in the blood, which increase the risks of heart disease.

Carbohydrates

The liver plays a central role in the control of the blood sugar level. It is able to do this by storing glucose from the diet and by synthesizing new glucose from non-carbohydrate sources such as amino acids and fatty acids.

If the liver is continuously metabolizing alcohol or drugs, the control of blood glucose becomes imprecise. This may result in periods of hypoglycaemia (low blood sugar level), which produces feelings of dizziness and faintness, and possibly blackouts or fainting. The problem may be aggravated if the pancreas is failing to produce insulin normally. Insulin is a key hormone in the control of blood glucose, and its absence results in diabetes.

Protein

A normal, healthy body maintains a balance between protein synthesis and degradation. Again, the liver is the main site for this protein metabolism. In an alcoholic or drug-detoxifying liver, protein degradation continues at an approx-imately normal rate. Protein synthesis, however, is poor, so that normal tissue repair is inefficient. End-products of protein metabolism are lost in the urine, with a state of protein deficiency slowly developing in the body.

Enzymes are inadequately produced; these include digestive enzymes and those involved in metabolism.

Water-soluble vitamins

The B complex vitamins are the ones most commonly lacking in alcoholics. Mixed B-complex deficiency may occur, involving nicotinic acid and riboflavin, and causing sore mouth and tongue, sore or gritty eyes, dermatitis, diarrhoea and psychological disturbance. There may also be a megaloblastic anaemia resulting from folic acid and vitamin B_{12} deficiencies; these occur due to loss of their enzymes or absorptive sites in the small intestine.

One of the most common single nutrient deficiencies is that of thiamine (vitamin B_1). This is required for alcohol metabolism and so needs are raised in an alcoholic.

If the intake is already low and increased thiamine is lost in vomit and urine, an acute thiamine deficiency may be precipitated. This may manifest as neurological disturbance affecting hands and feet, often with paralysis, making walking painful and difficult. More seriously, psychological disturbances with loss of memory and psychosis (known as Korsakoff's syndrome) may arise. Some of these patients do not recover on treatment.

Low vitamin C levels have also been reported in alcoholics and drug addicts, with bleeding gums and anaemia as the main signs. Poor vitamin C status may also increase susceptibility to infection, and cause delayed wound healing on injury.

Fat-soluble vitamins

Alcohol affects the fat-soluble vitamins less than it does the water-soluble vitamins, because there is a greater body reserve of the fat-soluble vitamins and no increased loss in the urine. On the other hand, all these vitamins require normal bile production for absorption and are stored in the liver. Thus, the status of some of the fat-soluble vitamins may become poor over a period of time.

Minerals

Zinc. Alcoholics may become zinc-depleted, as most of the body's zinc becomes directed towards alcohol oxidation as part of the enzyme used. Some of the consequences of poor zinc status include abnormalities of taste – which may contribute to a reduction of appetite, and delayed wound healing.

Electrolytes. Electrolytes such as potassium, magnesium and sodium may become unbalanced as a result of high levels or loss from the digestive tract in vomit and diarrhoea. This applies to both alcoholics and drug addicts. Severe depletion of potassium can cause cardiac arrest, so is very dangerous.

Iron. Alcoholics may run the risk of iron overload rather than deficiency. This is largely dependent on the nature of the drink taken, and the rest of the dietary intake.

Iron absorption is very carefully regulated in the small intestine to match the body's requirements (see Chapter 7). Alcohol breaks down this regulatory mechanism, allowing more iron to be absorbed. If the drink consumed contains iron, then large amounts of this mineral can be absorbed and accumulate in the body. The major iron-rich alcoholic beverages are cider and red wine.

If an alcoholic drinks spirits, and eats few foods containing iron (this is also likely in a drug addict), he or she is more likely to become iron-deficient, presenting with an anaemia. This may have a mixed clinical picture as it may be caused by both iron and B_{12}/folic acid deficiencies.

In summary, alcoholics and drug addicts place themselves at nutritional risk, by the effects of their addiction on their food intake, digestion and metabolism. Whenever possible, it is important that food intake is maintained to offset the harmful effects of the addiction. The use of supplements of multivitamins and protein can be beneficial when the opportunity arises for their administration.

Where a reasonable nutrition intake is maintained, adequate health can be sustained.

Poverty

Poverty and inadequte nutrition may be linked, although malnutrition is not an inevitable consequence of poverty.

In the West overt malnutrition is not often seen and may well be the result of a number of interacting factors. It is fairly well established that there are several diet-related diseases in the West; their incidence can be studied as an indicator of the effects of poverty on nutritional status and health.

A study of health and social class in Britain in 1980 found that still-births, congenital defects, and diseases of the cardiovascular and digestive systems exhibit a social class gradient, with the highest occurrence in the lowest social class.

Differences in food intake between the rich and poor

The National Food Survey in Britain describes average individual food and nutrient intakes and expenditure and provides useful information on income group differences in intakes.

Table 14.1 shows the foods whose intakes vary the most between the highest and lowest income households. The differences between the groups are compounded by the presence of children.

Nutritionally, the lower income diets are shown to be at risk of containing little dietary fibre, vitamin C, folic acid, vitamin E, zinc and too much sugar, compared with those of higher income groups. Fresh fruit and vegetables and fresh meat are the items most commonly omitted from the diet in a low-income household.

There is also a high prevalence of going without meals. One study found that 50% of adults and four in ten children reported often missing meals. Other studies have shown that it is frequently the mother in the household who misses meals, so that the father and children can have a greater share of the food available.

It has been recognized for many years that expenditure of food is one of the most 'elastic' items in the family outgoings. This means that when income is limited and other, fixed expenses have to be met, the food budget can be trimmed accordingly. Nevertheless, expenditure on food still represents 27% of the budget in the lowest income group (1985 figure, Family Expenditure Survey) and only 16% of the

Table 14.1 Differences in intakes of some foods between high and low income households in Britain (derived from National Food Survey data).

Compared with high-income households, people in low-income households eat considerably *more*:		Compared with high-income households, people in low-income households eat considerably *less*:
processed meat		cheese
eggs	} high in fat and sugar; nutrient-dilute	carcase meat
margarine		poultry
lard		fish
sugar		butter
jam		cooking oils
potatoes		fresh/frozen vegetables
canned vegetables (especially baked beans)	} relatively cheap and filling	fresh fruit
		brown/wholemeal bread
white bread		

budget of the highest income group. The *actual* amount of money spent was 38%
more in the top quarter of incomes compared with the lowest quarter.

The National Food Survey consistently demonstrates that the lowest income
groups actually obtain more nutrients per unit of money spent; thus the food
bought represents better nutrient value for money. Nevertheless, because of the
relatively small total amount of money available to spend on food, there is still a
considerably greater risk in the low-income groups of failing to meet the recommended levels for some of the nutrients.

Nutritional implications

Current dietary advice (described in Chapter 11) is for people to eat more fruit,
vegetables, pulses and wholegrain cereals, to reduce consumption of fatty meat,
choosing leaner cuts, poultry and fish, and to cut down on whole-fat dairy
products, replacing where necessary with reduced-fat alternatives.

Although both the high and low income groups eat similar total amounts of meat
products, closer analysis of the NFS data shows that more of the fatter meats and
meat products, which are cheaper, are eaten in the lower-income groups. The
higher-income groups chose more of the leaner carcase meats and poultry; these
are more expensive. These leaner meats provide less energy, so that the total
energy of a meal has to be made up with additional items, such as vegetables, pasta,
potatoes, bread, etc., further increasing the cost of the meal. A high-fat meat
product, such as a meat pie, needs few additional items to make it into a complete
meal – which makes it even more economical.

There is therefore little cost incentive for a family on a low budget to choose the
healthier, leaner meat. It makes better economic sense to buy the cheaper, more
filling meat product. A further advantage of the meat product is that it requires
little extra preparation and so is also economical in terms of cooking fuel.

Similar arguments hold for wholemeal cereal products which are currently more
expensive than the comparable refined products.

Fruit and vegetables are often viewed as luxury items – attractive and pleasant
to have in the diet, but not really essential for filling an empty stomach.

Food manufacturers are attempting to help the move towards more healthy
foods by providing an increasing variety of healthier alternatives. Unfortunately
they tend to be more expensive than the original versions. Even the convenience
foods are more costly, putting them beyond the reach of the poorer groups.

The trend in shopping habits and shopping provision is also an obstacle to
healthier eating for the poor. Local shops in the poorer neighbourhoods may stock
a limited range of foods, not including 'healthier' items for which the demand is
small. Therefore, if families want to buy these items, they may have to travel to a
more distant shop, adding to the cost. Out-of-town supermarkets sell a wide
selection of goods, offering a choice of healthier alternatives. Unfortunately those
on a low income can rarely afford to shop there, lacking transport and enough
money to make the trip worthwhile.

Inability to obtain a healthier diet is frustrating for some people on a low income.
Their inability to obtain healthier alternatives is by no means an indication of lack
of awareness or interest in the effects of food on their health. It simply reflects the
necessity to feed family members as economically as possible.

...t was actually costed and compared to the typical food ...income family (in 1986), the cost was 35% higher.

...cially at risk

...have been occasional cases reported in Britain of overt malnutrition in ...ren in the 1980s. However, the real extent of malnutrition in children is unknown. Information is based, for example, on studies of growth: these show that a significant proportion of poor children fall below the normal distribution for growth. The extent of the poor growth was highly correlated with the amount of money spent on food. In one London survey (in 1979), 11% of the children were mildly or moderately malnourished.

Specific nutrients that have been reported as low or lacking in groups of children include protein, iron, vitamin D, calcium and energy. These are nutrients whose inadequate intake may well result in poor physical development, poor dentition and anaemia, with associated lethargy.

School meals have been shown to make a more important contribution to the diets of these children than of children from higher income groups, whose out-of-school intakes are nutritionally more sound.

Young adults

The MAFF study in 1985 of the dietary habits of 15 to 25-year-olds in Britain showed that in the low-income groups there were low intakes of thiamine, ribo-flavin and calcium in both young men and women, together with low intakes of vitamin C in young men and of protein, nicotinic acid and fat in young women.

There are further studies reporting low iron and folic acid intakes among these women.

The implications are of concern, particularly as many of these young adults may become parents. Poor nutrition at conception may adversely affect development of the foetus. In addition, their inability to provide an adequate diet for themselves does not hold out much hope for the future diet of the children that may be born.

Women

Women form the majority of the poor in Britain; they include wage earners who receive low pay, almost two-thirds of the elderly population and nine-tenths of single-parent families. In families, women have been shown to go without food more often than men, to provide enough for the children. Low food intake in women reduces their opportunities for health. In pregnancy, when needs are increased, it may also affect the development of the baby. Studies in 1982 and 1986 have shown that poor pregnant women in Britain are consuming inadequate diets, falling up to 4.2 MJ per day short of the recommended intakes. These mothers have a higher than average incidence of low-birthweight babies.

Subsequently, the poorly nourished mother is less likely to breast feed success-fully. In a deprived environment there is a higher risk of infection for the baby who is bottle fed. The costs of bottle feeding are also higher; but without appropriate support, breast feeding is generally not undertaken in the lower income groups.

Elderly

Pensioners comprise almost 30% of the poorest people in Britain. Because appetite tends to decrease with age, yet nutrient needs remain relatively high, the diet of an elderly person should be nutrient-dense. Unfortunately many of the cheaper, more filling foods tend to have a lower nutrient density, thus placing the pensioner at risk of inadequate nutrition.

Ethnic minorities

As discussed earlier in this chapter, many immigrant groups prefer to eat foods typical of their own culture. These are generally more expensive and may be available only in more distant shops; thus travel costs further increase the total costs of the food.

Unemployment is particularly high among these communities; they may also have a high proportion of children and young people in the family group. All of these factors individually contribute to the risk of nutritional inadequacy; language problems may also restrict claims for benefit which could ease the poverty.

Disabled

At least two-thirds of the disabled population are estimated to be living at around the poverty level in Britain. For many, an adequate healthy diet may be crucial to their well-being.

The disability is likely to make access to shops difficult, so there may be greater dependence on local shops with perhaps a more limited choice and higher costs. This may make healthy diet an impossibility. Difficulties in food preparation or eating may further limit an intake restricted by poverty.

The homeless

The homeless who spend their nights in hostel or 'bed and breakfast' accommodation may have very little access to adequate cooking facilities, and are restricted to eating in cafés or preparing quick meals on a single-ring cooker in their rooms. In both cases, the overall food intake is a long way from the goals of a healthy diet.

Conclusion

In summary, poverty in the West has been shown to result in or increase the risk of malnutrition. The poor may have the knowledge and the desire to consume a healthful diet as currently recommended; unfortunately economic pressures on their limited finances prevent them from achieving this. Groups particularly at risk have been identified, and include those whose access to food is further limited by age, language barriers or disability.

15

Adverse Reactions to Food and Unorthodox Diets

During recent years there has been a considerable growth of interest in adverse reactions to food. To many, all reactions to food are seen as 'food allergy'. This term, however, has a precise meaning which has been widely misunderstood.

Food allergy is a form of food intolerance that causes reproducible symptoms and includes abnormal immunological reactions to the food.

The normal diet contains a variety of substances that stimulate immune responses (allergens). These are usually proteins, or simple chemicals bound to proteins. In normal individuals, these allergens induce immune responses; they are usually detected as serum antibodies. Therefore the detection of serum antibody to a given allergen does not imply that the allergen is implicated in disease. A food allergy only arises when the immune response produces *abnormal* or pathological changes in the gut or other sites.

Food intolerance is a more general term, and is applied to all reproducible adverse reactions to food that are not psychologically based. As well as food allergy, it includes reactions to food additives, natural components of foods, microorganisms and their products, and phenomena due to inborn errors. In this last group are included enzyme deficiencies causing disorders of metabolism and gluten sensitivity (coeliac disease). None of these produces an immunological response, and cannot therefore be termed food allergy.

Food aversion occurs when a food is avoided for psychological reasons, or when physical reactions are produced by the emotions, rather than the food itself. This latter behaviour may be mistakenly interpreted as a true food allergy by the subject, with subsequent avoidance of foods. In extreme cases this can lead to a very unbalanced diet.

Prevalence

Food intolerance is extremely difficult to study epidemiologically. There is an almost limitless number of foodstuffs and additives that could provoke a response. The symptoms produced are extremely diverse and may occur immediately after exposure to the food, or after some considerable period. The testing for food allergy in large numbers of people is laborious and the tests themselves may not be particularly sensitive. Confirming the diagnosis in an individual is time-consuming and involves considerable interference with the subject's life.

Consequently, figures which are quoted for prevalence are very variable. The Royal College of Physicians in 1984 quoted 0.3 to 2% of children as suffering from dietary intolerance. Further, a 0.03 to 0.1% prevalence of food additive intolerance has been reported by the Commission of European Communities.

Clinical presentation

Reactions to food are enormously diverse and variable in severity. Broadly, the symptoms fall into two categories: immediate, and delayed in onset. The symptoms may be general and severe enough to be life-threatening; this is called *anaphylaxis*.

More commonly, they affect the following tissues and systems:

(1) *Gastrointestinal system*. Symptoms include mouth tingling or swelling, abdominal pain, bloating of the abdomen, vomiting and diarrhoea, or constipation.

In chronic intolerance, there can be bleeding or loss of plasma protein into the gut lumen with damage to the gut mucosa.

(2) *Skin*. Dermatitis, urticaria, angioedema and eczema are common consequences.

(3) *Respiratory system*. Rhinitis and asthma (including wheezing, breathlessness).

(4) *Central-nervous system*. Migraine; possibly some behavioural abnormalities (including schizophrenia, depression and hyperactivity) but the evidence for these is far from conclusive.

The mechanisms involved

The alimentary tract can absorb a certain amount of antigenic material (usually protein), which passes into the lymphatic system and blood, and stimulates the immune system. In some individuals with a predisposition to producing antibodies of the immunoglobulin E (IgE) class, allergen-specific IgE is produced. This IgE attaches to mast cells in the tissues, particularly in the skin, respiratory system and digestive tract, where it reacts with the allergens. The mast cells release a variety of chemical mediators, such as histamine and prostaglandins, which can cause the immediate hypersensitivity reactions. These symptoms can include:

(1) dilation of small blood vessels (redness);
(2) increased permeability of blood vessels (swelling);
(3) contraction of smooth muscle in the airways (breathing difficulties) or intestines (causing pain);
(4) stimulation of nerve endings in the skin (itching and pain).

The immune complexes may also circulate in the blood, attached to serum antibodies. They are successfully removed in a normal individual, but in an allergic person they can be carried to the tissues causing a further inflammatory response.

The absorption of allergens is normally prevented by secretory immunoglobulin A (IgA) in the gut, which can coat microorganisms and food antigens. IgA deficiency is normal in the first months of life, thus the risk of developing allergies to foods is greater at this time. Avoidance of contact with potential allergens is important at this age, especially where there is a family history of allergy. This can significantly reduce later development of allergies. Breast feeding also offers some protection against allergy development, possibly due to the IgA present in human milk.

Diagnosis

The diagnosis of food intolerance must be performed according to strict criteria. Three approaches may be used:

(1) Clinical assessment.
(2) Dietary manipulation.
(3) Laboratory tests.

Clinical assessment

This uses the medical history of the subject to indicate if there is a likelihood of a food intolerance. In some cases the link with food may be obvious, if the reaction is associated with meals. However, delayed reactions may be difficult to associate with eating.

A food diary kept over a period of two or three weeks is likely to identify foods that appear frequently and may be the cause of the intolerance.

Dietary manipulation

Where no particular foods are suspected an 'elimination diet' of varying rigour is introduced. The most severe allows only lamb, pears and bottled spring water for five days. This diet should be supervised, and *not* undertaken by the person of their own accord. If an improvement occurs, a food intolerance may be suspected. Individual foods or groups of related foods may then gradually be reintroduced, and reactions noted. Care should be exercised here as severe reactions can occur.

The testing procedure may be performed 'blind'. This means that neither the subject nor the doctor are aware of the nature of the test food, and whether it is 'safe'. Presenting the subject with a food to which he considers himself allergic may itself precipitate a reaction. Considerable ingenuity may be necessary to make the food testing truly 'blind'.

Where several foods are the cause of sensitivity the testing procedure may take several weeks, or even months.

If the testing is done at home, the subject may be advised to avoid particular foods and record symptoms. With common foods such as eggs, milk or wheat, considerable numbers of foods have to be omitted, which can be very difficult.

Laboratory tests

The subject may be skin-tested with purified extracts of the food; the size of the weal developing on the skin being used to assess reactivity. Applying drops of the food extract under the tongue and measuring the pulse rate is an alternative method of testing. Neither of these alone can diagnose allergy, and dietary challenge must also be used.

Immunological tests include the measurement of raised IgE levels in the serum (RAST), but even this may give a negative result in some forms of food allergy, and not necessarily agree with clinical symptoms.

Examination of tissue samples from the intestinal mucosa after the elimination of suspect foods and on their reintroduction can provide further evidence.

Foods causing intolerance

Any food can be considered allergenic, but some appear to cause reactions more commonly than others. The same food may produce different symptoms in different individuals. The foods most commonly causing sensitivity include eggs, milk, wheat, fish, pork, bacon, peanuts, rice, cheese, soya, yeast, nuts and tomatoes. Often a person may be allergic to more than one food item.

Pharmacological reactions

Some food intolerance reactions are due to the presence of pharmacologically active agents in food. For example, caffeine has been reported as a cause of food reaction in some people. Cheese, wine, bananas, yeast extract, avocados, chocolate and oranges, all of which contain amines such as histamine, may produce intolerance symptoms.

Usually the reaction occurs after a quite large ingestion of the offending substance, unlike a true food allergy, where even a small intake can trigger a reaction.

Other food constituents may cause the release of neurotransmitter substances in the brain, which can result in behavioural or mood changes. However, this area still needs further investigation.

Food additives

There are an increasing number of reports claiming that clinical reactions including urticaria, angioedema and asthma, as well as hyperactivity in children, are caused by particular food additives. Those mentioned most commonly include colouring agents such as tartrazine, and antioxidants such as BHT (butylated hydroxytoluene) and BHA (butylated hydroxyanisole).

The diagnosis of these reactions is extremely difficult, as no immunological effect is involved. In addition, additives are rarely consumed singly, so individual reactions are difficult to identify.

Considerable attention has been given to the possible association between additives and *hyperactivity* in children. The theory originated with Feingold in 1973, who reported that ingestion of artificial food additives (colours and flavours) and naturally occurring salicylates in foods caused hyperactivity and learning disabilities in children. The elimination of all these substances from the diet was claimed by Feingold to produce a 'full response' in 50% of hyperactive, learning-disabled children.

One of the major problems in this area is that hyperactivity is an ill-defined state, and can result from a variety of causes. This confusion results in differing figures for its prevalence, from 0.09% in the UK up to 5% in the USA. As a result, Feingold's results have not been repeated successfully in properly controlled studies. Indeed, results from small controlled studies have been conflicting.

Challenging the child with artificial colours has not necessarily provoked a response, and there have even been differences in teachers' and parents' assessments of the same children. These problems highlight some of the difficulties of study in this area.

Treatment of food intolerance

As most food allergens occur in a limited number of foods, it should be possible to eliminate these from the diet, once the allergen has been identified. This does require professional advice from a dietitian, as few people know enough about the composition of food and nutritional needs to ensure a well-balanced diet. In addition, some common allergens may occur in manufactured food, where their presence may not be suspected. Incorrect advice from ill-informed people may actually lead to nutritional problems, rather than resolving them.

Food intolerance is not necessarily a permanent condition, so that avoidance of the allergen for a period of time may ultimately allow its reintroduction, at least in small amounts. Young children, in particular, sometimes 'grow out of' food intolerances, presumably as the gut matures and becomes less permeable to allergens.

More comprehensive food labelling allows the consumer to more readily identify foods containing unsafe substances. Sufferers from coeliac disease, who must avoid gluten from wheat, can obtain lists of safe foods from the Coeliac Society. Many such foods carry the 'crossed grains' symbol, indicating their safety for coeliacs.

Illness and food allergy

Food allergy has been suggested as a cause of various common illnesses. These are considered briefly.

Atopic eczema

Atopic eczema is an inflammatory, itchy skin disorder, present in babies and children. It tends to run in families and is often also associated with hayfever and asthma.

The eczema can be exacerbated by factors such as stress, contact with animals and food intolerance. Only some sufferers have raised IgE levels in the blood. The use of elimination diets has met with some success; removal of eggs and milk has been most successful. If a child responds to such a 'safe' diet, it is important to ensure an adequate intake of calcium, vitamins A and D. Also, such a diet may be very difficult for a child to keep to.

Breast feeding a child at risk of eczema (indicated by the family history) may reduce the likelihood of the disease developing. The use of soya or goat's milk has not been shown to lessen the risk of allergy; goat's milk is nutritionally inadequate for children under 6 months.

Migraine

Migraine is a disorder characterized by recurrent attacks of headaches and visual symptoms, of varying intensity and duration, occasionally also with nausea and vomiting. The condition often runs in families. However, there is controversy as to whether migraine is the result of a true food allergy or a food intolerance. Elimination diets both for children and adults have identified specific foods which trigger headaches in some individuals. In adults, the commonest triggering foods were found to be wheat, oranges, eggs, tea, coffee, chocolate, milk, beef, mushrooms and peas. Among children, headaches were triggered with milk, egg, chocolate, oranges and wheat. Reactions to more than one food were common.

Skin-prick testing in the children did not predict trigger foods. In addition, when the children were tested in a 'blind' study with the foods, only 65% reacted with headaches. No immunological mechanism could be detected.

An alternative suggestion for the mechanism of migraine is that many of the triggering foods contain tyramine, a derivative of the amino acid tyrosine. Tyramine is usually broken down in the body by the enzyme monoamine oxidase; if this is defective, tyramine may build up in the blood. Giving tyramine to migraine sufferers does trigger headache.

It is possible that the abnormal amine response is part of a true food allergy, but at present, migraine cannot strictly be described as such.

Multiple sclerosis

Multiple sclerosis is a degenerative disease of the nervous system, affecting 1.2 per 1000 adults in the UK. At present there is no cure for the disease; many dietary treatments have been proposed, including supplementation with sunflower or evening primrose oil, or the avoidance of specific foods, such as milk or gluten.

However, as yet none of these treatments has been found to give any measurable benefit to sufferers. It is unlikely that a food intolerance is involved.

Rheumatoid arthritis

Rheumatoid arthritis is a disease of the connective tissue around the joints, especially in the hands and fingers, but it can affect the whole body. The joints become inflamed and this may trigger muscle spasms, which ultimately deform the joint. The cause of rheumatoid arthritis is unknown, although it is suggested that it may be an autoimmune disease, in which the patient develops antibodies to his or her own tissues, possibly to circulating prostaglandins.

Some sufferers claim benefit from a fairly strict exclusion diet, called the Dong Diet. It was initially developed by Dr Dong, who himself suffered from arthritis. The diet eliminates dairy produce, beef, lamb, pork, fruit, spices, alcohol and chemical additives, including preservatives. Foods that are permitted include fish, chicken, vegetables, rice, potatoes and plain bread (without additives and preservatives). Studies of arthritic patients who eliminate certain foods from their diet have noted some benefits in terms of symptom relief; the disease, however, is not 'cured'.

We are a long way from understanding this condition, or the possible role of food intolerance in its symptoms.

Diet and cancer therapy

Treatment of cancer by traditional methods includes surgery, radiotherapy and chemotherapy. Many people are afraid of these treatments, perceiving them as painful, disfiguring and with unpleasant side effects.

It is important to remember that a patient undergoing cancer therapy should be in as good a nutritional state as the illness will permit. It is generally recognized that treatment is both more effective and better tolerated in such circumstances.

However, this may be difficult to achieve, as tumours and treatments can affect appetite and taste as well as the psychological desire to eat. Digestive and absorptive processes may be inefficient if the gastrointestinal tract is affected; some of the treatments can cause severe diarrhoea and thus reduce absorption. Finally, the metabolism may be abnormal, with the tumour diverting nutrients for its own growth and thus depriving healthy tissues. In addition, the metabolic rate may be above normal, actually increasing nutritional needs.

Some cancer sufferers turn to unorthodox forms of treatment, either because of uncertainty about traditional therapy, or from a positive desire to become more actively involved in their own treatment. In addition, alternative therapy focuses on the patient as a whole, rather than just the disease, considering both the psychological and physical aspects of the patient. This approach is termed 'holistic', and occurs in many of the alternative therapies.

Several alternative forms of cancer therapy have been promoted, which include dietary modification. These date from as far back as the 1940s. In recent years the programme that has gained publicity in Britain is that of the Cancer Help Centre in Bristol, devised by Dr Forbes. Other centres have also been established using the Bristol system.

Briefly, the programme includes diet, metabolic therapy, self-healing, psychotherapy and healing, in a 'total therapy' approach to treating cancer. The diet aims to create conditions in the body that will destroy the cancer and restore the body's natural immunity, which has been weakened by the poor diet.

The diet itself is vegetarian and low in protein, with a large proportion (at least 70%) of the food being consumed raw. This is to enable the vitamins and enzymes contained in it to be delivered unchanged to the patient. The enzymes are believed to be needed to break down the protein coat of the cancer cells. Protein intake is also low, to spare the body's protein-digesting enzymes for cancer cell destruction, (this does not seem probable, from current physiological knowledge).

In addition, the diet permits cereals and pulses; but meat, dairy products and all processed foods, – which may contain undesirable additives and lack 'vital' ingredients – are forbidden. Tea and coffee, which contain stimulants such as caffeine, are also forbidden, although alcohol is allowed in small quantities.

This diet is extremely bulky, and for a patient with possibly advanced cancer whose appetite is small, it is unlikely to provide adequate essential nutrients. In addition, a malnourished patient will have difficulty absorbing many nutrients if the gut mucosa is damaged. Hence the diet may aggravate a malnourished state. On the other hand, preparation of food and the patient's own involvement in the treatment provide a psychological benefit. Other aspects of the therapy also provide psychological support for the patients.

Many nutritional supplements are taken, some orthodox, others quite unorthodox. There are anecdotal case reports of the effectiveness of the treatment, however, a true scientific evaluation has not been made. Some of the claims for the mechanisms of action of the diet, and the rationale behind the dietary therapy, do not fit current scientific knowledge.

However, while some patients continue to benefit from this therapy, it should not be completely dismissed.

Weight-reducing diets

Overweight and obesity are major problems in the West, and increasingly among the wealthy in certain Third World countries. For many people excess weight is a persistent problem, despite their efforts at weight loss.

A major industry has grown up aiming to help people in their quest for weight loss. Much of the publicity and advice suggests that weight loss can be easy, quick and permanent, if only the individual uses 'Formula A' or follows 'Diet B'. The lack of long-term success is evidence that most of these promises are meaningless.

The fundamental (and only) way to reduce weight is to reduce energy intake below the level of energy output. This should ideally be achieved by changes in both. If the energy output is sufficiently increased by greater physical activity, then reduction in energy intake need not be great. In this way a balanced diet can be maintained.

The major problem with many diet plans and special 'slimming foods' is that they take little account of the subject's usual eating habits or nutritional needs. As a result, slimmers see themselves as being 'on a diet', and look forward to the day the diet ends, so that they can return to their normal eating. The usual result of this is that weight is regained and the slimming diet has to start again.

Many overweight people spend decades in this way, losing and regaining weight and always looking for the ultimate diet, which will make the weight loss permanent. It is not surprising that many hundreds of diets have been devised.

Recently, a number of 'very low calorie diets' have been marketed. These contain a complete liquid-formula meal, providing less than 2.5 MJ/day, designed for rapid weight loss. Most of those sold in the UK provide 1.3 to 1.4 MJ/day. The formula contains approximately 30 g of protein and 30 to 40 g of carbohydrate, with minimal amounts of fat. Vitamins and minerals are included to meet recommended intakes; the mixture is flavoured to increase palatability.

Early formulations of these diets were deficient in essential amino acids and resulted in over 50 sudden deaths in the USA. However, with a better nutritional balance and the addition of some carbohydrate, they are now considered safe for up to 4 weeks' use.

Weight loss on these diets averages 1.5 kg per week, if all meals are replaced to give a daily intake of 1.35 MJ. It is reported that people using the diets do not feel hungry; this may be due to the raised levels of ketones in the blood, which cause a loss of appetite.

Reported side effects include gastrointestinal upsets, such as nausea and diarrhoea, as well as constipation. Some hair loss, gout and heartbeat irregularities have also been reported.

A major concern for slimmers is the maintenance of weight loss. The use of very low calorie diets does not retrain the appetite or change eating habits; a return to normal eating is therefore likely to result in weight regain. Studies show that this is indeed the case, with some 85% of subjects regaining at least 50% of their lost weight. One possible factor in the weight gain is the loss of lean body mass while on the diet. This leads to a fall in basal metabolic rate and thence the energy requirement. If lean body mass is not regained, the metabolic rate remains depressed, resulting in easier weight gain.

Despite these drawbacks, very low calorie diets have become popular. They are used both clinically in the very overweight to start the weight loss process, and also by the only slightly overweight to lose weight for a special occasion. The long-term consequences of such manipulation of body weight and composition remain a possible problem for the future.

16
Diet and Dental Health

There are two main diseases affecting the teeth and gums for which a relationship with the diet has been suggested. These are dental caries, and periodontal (gum) disease.

Dental caries

Dental caries is the major disease, affecting the tooth itself; it progressively destroys the tooth, causing pain and infection and, if unchecked, leads to the loss of the tooth. It is said to be one of the most common diseases of mankind.

Periodontal disease

Periodontal disease takes several forms. It may affect the gums or gingival margins (gingivitis), or the deeper tissues (periodontitis). The latter involves gradual loss of bone, which eventually leads to looseness and loss of teeth. Most children have some gingivitis, of varying severity. Periodontitis affects a small number of teenagers and a significant proportion of adults. Prevention of periodontitis can result in retention of the teeth for as long as possible.

Incidence of dental disease

Ancient populations had low prevalence of dental disease; this began to increase with the development of civilization. A similar trend has been seen this century in primitive populations exposed to western influences. For example, the Eskimos in Greenland have exhibited a rise in caries prevalence during the period from 1914 to 1945; the extent of caries has been related to their proximity to main trading stations.

Since the 1970s reductions in the occurrence of dental caries of between 35 to 50% in children have been noted in many western countries. There is still debate as to the exact causes of this reversal in the upward trend. Possible reasons are discussed later in this chapter.

In the UK, the number of adults with active decay in 1978 had fallen to 59%, from 64% in 1968; in addition 29% of the population in 1979 had no natural teeth, compared with 37% in 1968. In 1978 nearly half of the 5-year-olds in Britain had some signs of decay.

In Third World populations, among rural dwellers and those eating traditional diets, caries remains a relatively minor problem, but in urban populations,

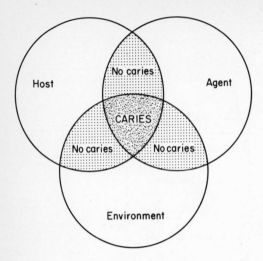

Fig. 16.1   Parameters contributing to tooth decay.

exposed to westernizing influences, prevalence has increased rapidly. This has been attributed to the increased availability and use of sugar and refined flours, and foods prepared from them. These types of foods have prestige value, being associated with affluence; yet the problem that such foods can bring is rarely recognized.

Strictly speaking dental decay is not a dietary disease, but one that is of microbial origin. In order for tooth decay to occur, three parameters must occur simultaneously (see Fig. 16.1). A change in any of the three parameters can alter the severity of decay, either to decrease or increase it.

Agent

The presence of *Streptococcus mutans*, the major bacterial species believed to be responsible for the production of acids in the mouth, is not thought to be related to dietary intake or status. However, it is suggested that the activity of the bacterial enzymes may be reduced by the presence of fluoride ions (this is discussed later).

Host: the tooth and its susceptibility

The major parts of a tooth are illustrated in Fig. 16.2.

Human teeth are formed over a limited period of time, during development in the womb and the first years of life. Tooth formation may be adversely affected by factors such as malnutrition and infections. The teeth, once mineralized, have no mechanisms for repair, and any disturbances in their formation will be apparent as irreversible damage in the part of the tooth corresponding to the stage of development. These damaged teeth are more susceptible to attack and caries formation.

Reduction of enamel thickness (hypoplasia) has been found in malnourished children and correlates with low socio-economic status. The precise nutritional deficiency resulting in hypoplasia has not been identified with certainty. Vitamin

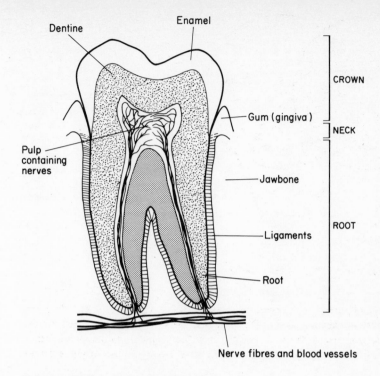

Fig. 16.2 The main parts of a typical tooth.

D deficiency and associated low blood calcium levels around birth may be responsible. Premature and low-birthweight infants are particularly at risk, as they tend to have low vitamin D status. Vitamin A and C deficiencies may also be involved. Fluoride is the most important trace element involved in the development of caries-resistant teeth.

Environment

The oral environment provides the raw materials to be fermented into acid by bacteria, thus creating conditions for caries development. *Streptococcus mutans* rapidly ferments dietary sucrose, producing acid in the mouth within minutes of sugar ingestion. From simple dietary carbohydrates, *S. mutans* also produces long-chain polysaccharides (polyglucans) that adhere to the teeth in the form of plaque. The polysaccharides are metabolized over a period of time by the bacteria to organic acids such as citric and pyruvic acids. These acids then solubilize and dissolve the hydroxyapatite of the tooth enamel.

The process of tooth dissolution is reversible, particularly in the early stages of attack. Fluoride in the mouth environment is thought to assist in mineral redeposition within the tissue. Further, dietary fibre may supply increased phosphate, which also promotes remineralization.

Plaque is also the major cause of periodontal disease. Although the bacteria in

Table 16.1 The influence of dietary factors in caries production via agent, environment and host.

	Promoting factors	Reducing factors
Agent	?	Fluoride
Environment	Dietary carbohydrate, especially sugars	Fluoride
		Phosphate
Host	•? Low calcium/vitamin D during tooth development	Fluoride
	? General malnutrition	
	? Vitamin A deficiency	
	? Vitamin C deficiency	

plaque do not invade the gum tissues directly, they do produce a number of substances that can cause inflammation of the gums. The most effective way of removing plaque is by tooth brushing.

Thus, dietary factors influence caries production through action on the agent, environment and host (see Table 16.1).

Dietary factors inhibiting decay

Fluoride

It has been appreciated for almost half a century that an optimum level of fluoride ions present in the diet during the period of tooth development causes a 50% or greater reduction in dental caries, compared with controls. Fluoride is believed to act in several ways.

(1) Fluoride strengthens teeth by converting hydroxyapatite crystals in the enamel to the less soluble fluorapatite.

(2) Remineralization of eroded enamel is enhanced by the presence of fluoride, probably by the stimulation of osteoblast cells.

(3) The presence of fluoride in the environment of the tooth also inhibits the metabolism of *Streptococcus mutans*, thereby reducing its ability to form acids and plaque.

(4) Fluoride present in the mouth can enter the outer enamel layers of the teeth, producing a higher content there than in the underlying dentine, with associated greater resistance to acid.

The major route by which fluoride is incorporated in the diet is via the drinking water. If the entire period of tooth development is to be encompassed, fluoride should be available from birth to the age of fourteen years.

Since 1944, fluoridation (the controlled addition of fluoride as part of the water treatment system) at 1 mg/l (or 1 ppm) has been introduced in many countries of the world. More than 230 million people in over 40 countries, including 100 million in the USA, drink fluoridated water. Over a hundred reports from all parts of the world have been published since 1951 supporting the original observations on the effectiveness of fluoridation. The desirability of water fluoridation has been endorsed by many national and international bodies, such as the (British) Royal College of Physicians and the World Health Organization. Since fluoridation was first introduced, allegations have been made that it causes cancer, mongolism, congenital malformation, cardiovascular deaths and allergies. None of these has been shown to have any association with fluoridation. The only side effect which may be encountered is a mild dental fluorosis, with patches on the enamel, which has been found where fluoride concentrations in the water exceed 2 to 3 mg/l. The costs of fluoridation of water supplies are very low; far less than the cost of dental treatment for teeth affected by caries.

Apart from this one possible side effect, there is an additional possible benefit in a reduced incidence of osteoporosis in fluoridated areas. Indeed, fluoride supplements have been used in treatment of osteoporosis.

Alternative routes of administering fluoride have been proposed and used in some studies. These avoid the problem of administering fluoride to people who feel it is their right to refuse what they perceive as 'mass medication'.

Fluoridated milk. The provision of fluoridated milk was first proposed in 1956. The major advantage is that fluoride is added to a staple food for children and that its consumption, being voluntary, can be confined to the most important group. Generally, the fluoridated milk is provided in school. Results obtained have generally been comparable with those of water fluoridation.

Fluoride supplements (taken in drops or tablets). These supplements are available for use by people who have no access to fluoridated water. Ideally the use of such supplements should begin from birth, to cover the whole of the tooth mineralization period. It is important to note that some infant milk formulae may already contain fluoride and thus supplementation may not be necessary.

The main problem with the use of fluoride supplements is the high degree of motivation required by the consumer; a conscious effort is required to maintain daily intake. There is also a risk of accidental poisoning if a large number of tablets are taken.

Topical fluoride. This refers to the application of fluoride to the tooth surface, rather than its ingestion. It has been established that fluoride in contact with the surface of the tooth does provide remineralization of the tooth enamel and reduces the incidence of dental caries. Dentists can apply fluoride solution or gel to children's teeth as part of a caries prevention programme, although this is a relatively expensive procedure.

Fluoride-containing toothpaste is widely available in many countries. In the UK in 1980 it accounted for 96% of the toothpaste available. In addition to the effects in the mouth, there is also a possibility that some of the fluoride in the toothpaste is actually ingested, as young children have a tendency to swallow toothpaste while tooth brushing; a small systemic effect may thus take place.

In summary, fluoride has been shown to reduce dental caries significantly. The best effects, with 50% or greater reductions, are obtained with fluoridated water (or naturally occurring fluoride-containing water supplies). This is also by far the most cost-effective method of fluoride administration. All other schemes are either intermittent or dependent on a high degree of motivation, and all are considerably more expensive.

Phosphate

The presence of phosphates in the dental plaque is said to favour remineralization rather than demineralization. Calcium glycerophosphate has been used as an additive to some fluoride toothpastes, to enhance the effects of the fluoride ion.

It is also suggested that the beneficial effects of dietary fibre on teeth may in part be mediated by the phosphate present in them. In particular phytate (inositol-6-phosphate) may release some phosphate into the mouth during chewing, thus enhancing the remineralization effect.

Dietary factors promoting decay

Carbohydrates

This is the dietary group most firmly implicated in the aetiology of dental caries. Evidence for the involvement of carbohydrates – particularly sugar – in dental caries comes from a large number of different types of studies.

(1) *Historical records* of dietary change show increases in dental disease with the introduction of sugar, and reductions when sugar was rationed and less refined cereal eaten, as in wartime in the UK.

(2) *Dietary manipulation in human studies*. The best known of the experimental studies on the effects of sugar on teeth was performed in Vipeholm (Sweden) in 1954. Subjects were allowed to eat sugar at meal times only, or freely throughout the day, and in liquid or dry forms. The greatest amount of caries occurred in subjects eating sugar between meals, and especially in the form of solid or 'sticky' sugar (like toffees). Sugar with meals had little cariogenic effect.

This study provided evidence to show that it is not simply the amount of sugar consumed that is important in decay, but also the form and frequency. Generally, sugar eaten as part of a meal is less cariogenic than that eaten between meals. Prolonged contact of sugar with teeth is most damaging.

(3) *Avoidance of sugar*. Individuals who have hereditary fructose intolerance and therefore avoid all foods containing sucrose (or fructose), such as sweets, cakes, pastries, have a dental caries prevalence of only 10%.

The daily use of as little as two sticks of sugar-containing chewing gum by children can produce a detectable increase of dental caries. However, substitution of the sugar with xylitol in chewing gum resulted in no new occurrence of caries. The use of xylitol as a substitute for sugar in some foods may thus inhibit the formation of new carious lesions and may also have a positive anticariogenic effect.

Relative cariogenicity of foods

The pH below which enamel demineralization begins has been called the 'critical pH'; it has been shown to be around 5.5.

The ability of a food item to cause low pH values in plaque is the major factor in determining its cariogenic potential. Careful measurement of pH changes in the mouth following the eating of a large variety of foods has identified dietary factors and foods of varying cariogenic potential. Some of these foods are listed in Table 16.2.

In Switzerland, it is permitted to label nonacidogenic products as 'safe for teeth'. This is the only country which has so far made this positive effort towards dental health promotion.

Table 16.2 Relative cariogenicity of some dietary factors and foods, based on acid-producing potential in the mouth.

	Most acidogenic	Moderately acidogenic	Non-acidogenic
Dietary factors	Sucrose Fructose Glucose Maltose	Galactose Lactose Starch	Xylitol Mannitol Sorbitol
Foods	Boiled sweets Toffees	Apples Chocolates Bananas	Peanuts Crisps Dried apples Dried apricots Fresh oranges Cheese Eggs

Although it is possible to identify particular foods which have marked or minor effects on the oral pH, the results of eating combinations of food in meals, with accompanying drinks, may be quite different. It is only when 'acid-producing' or 'safe' foods are eaten alone that the actual changes in the mouth can be predicted.

One group of sugar-containing items that has recently come under scrutiny is medicines, in particular those in liquid formulations. Many of these are designed for use in children, yet their sugar content in some cases reaches 60 to 70%. In addition, many products like cough syrups or throat lozenges are available without prescription, and may be consumed frequently and regularly by all age groups.

In summary, sucrose and the simple carbohydrates are strongly implicated in dental caries. Evidence is available from a number of studies employing differing approaches.

Measurements of actual acid production on the mouth after eating have identi-fied a number of foods which are apparently 'safe for teeth'. In addition, studies with xylitol and related substances have found these to be noncariogenic. It is clear, however, that the pattern, frequency and the nature of the sucrose consumed are as important in determining the subsequent development of caries, as the absolute quantity.

Dental health education

The messages of dental health education can be stated fairly simply.

(1) *Fluoridation* is the single most important measure for improving the dental health of the whole community. Where fluoridation is not available, fluoride drops, tablets or application by the dentist should be used.

(2) *Restriction of quantity and frequency of sucrose intake.* The number of times per day that the teeth are exposed to sugar is one of the major factors determining the rate of dental decay. If sugar intake is confined to mealtimes, the harmful effects of sugar are reduced. In particular, sugar in a 'sticky' form should be avoided.

(3) *Regular brushing with fluoride toothpaste.* Clean teeth and gums every day, using a fluoride toothpaste. Brushing the teeth disturbs and removes plaque, if done thoroughly. Many people's normal tooth-cleaning procedures leave behind

considerable amounts of plaque. The use of a fluoride toothpaste reduces the solubility of the outer enamel layers and allows the process of remineralization.

Trends in dental health point to an improvement in recent years. This has occurred both in fluoridated and unfluoridated regions, but dental health remains better where the water supply is fluoridated. The use of fluoride in toothpastes has become widespread in some countries. In the UK, almost all toothpaste sold is fluoridated. In France, only a small proportion of toothpaste is fluoridated and dental health improvements have been much less. In Japan, where fluoride toothpaste is almost unknown, caries has not been reduced at all.

There has also been a gradual fall in the annual sugar consumption in Britain, from 46.3 kg per person in 1970 to 37.9 kg per person in 1980. This is still well above the level of 15 kg per person per year which is suggested as the upper level for sugar consumption to prevent caries in most of the population (if fluoride toothpaste is used).

The fall in sugar intake has been accompanied by some beneficial changes in infant feeding patterns. For example, the practice of adding sugar to bottle feeds and the use of comforters dipped in or filled with sugary solutions has declined. In addition, vitamin C supplements for infants and children, which used to be given in a sugary syrup, are now dispensed as drops.

Processed baby foods have also followed the trend of reducing sugar contents.

However, dental decay still remains a problem, particularly among the poorer and disadvantaged sections of society. It has been described as a form of malnutrition, with a tendency for children presenting with caries to be below average weight. This suggests that these children may be consuming diets that provide energy but not nutrients, and are therefore malnourished.

This preventable condition requires attention to diet, adequate dental hygiene and fluoridation for prevention to succeed.

17
Nutrition and Public Health

This chapter reviews some of the links that have been described between nutrition and 'western diseases'. Some of these have been discussed in earlier chapters, in the context of specific nutrients, or as part of the advice for healthier eating.

The information is consolidated here, giving a more complete picture of the role of nutrition in major western diseases.

Coronary heart disease

Coronary heart disease is one of the major causes of death in the western world; in Britain it is the leading cause of death. Mortality from cardiovascular disease has been declining since the mid-1970s in many western countries, but the UK mortality rates have only very recently started to fall, and are therefore some of the highest in the world. Epidemiological research points to an association between cardiovascular disease and nutrition, but cannot confirm a causal relationship. Neither is it possible to explain fully the observed reductions in heart disease incidence.

The major difficulty in establishing such a relationship lies in the multifactorial nature of the disease. This means that many features may increase the likelihood of a person's developing heart disease. The existence of just one or two risk factors may appear to have little effect; however, the more risk factors there are present, the greater the risk of the disease.

Three major risk factors have been identified.

(1) *Raised blood lipid levels*. The most studied of these has been the cholesterol level.

(2) *Cigarette smoking*. Persuading at-risk subjects to stop smoking can result in a significant reduction of their heart disease risk.

(3) *Raised blood pressure*. Individuals with a raised arterial blood pressure have a greater risk of both coronary heart disease and stroke. Reduction of blood pressure, by drug treatment, weight loss or dietary modification, is likely therefore to be of benefit.

Other risk factors also operate:

(4) *Age and sex*. Men are at greater risk than women below the age of 60 years; it has been suggested that the female hormones are protective prior to the menopause. The occurrence of heart disease increases with age; the median age of death from cardiovascular disease is 74 years in England and Wales.

(5) *Social class*. Men in social classes I and II (the professional classes) have a

lower than average risk of death from coronary heart disease, while those from social class V have a higher than average risk. The traditional view of the 'stressed businessman' as the one at greatest risk is not supported by the mortality statistics.

The recent reduction in heart disease mortality in the UK has been much greater in the higher social classes, thus widening the gap.

(6) *Family history*. There is evidence that heart disease risk is greater in relatives of individuals who already exhibit the disease. This may relate to a genetic difference in the handling of fats in the body.

(7) *Physical activity*. Exercise has been promoted as desirable in the reduction of heart disease risk, based on studies that show lower mortality in those who undertake some form of physical exercise, compared with sedentary controls. The mechanisms involved are unclear and may include several factors, such as changes in blood lipids, the levels of clotting factors in the blood or the density of capillaries in the tissues.

(8) *Obesity*. Studies have failed to find a direct effect of overweight on heart disease risk. However, when body fat distribution has been taken into account, and subjects divided into 'apples' (abdominal obesity) and 'pears' (peripheral obesity), a relationship with heart disease is seen for 'apples'. In addition, obesity is frequently associated with raised blood pressure, raised blood lipid levels, and non-insulin-dependent diabetes mellitus. All of these may independently increase the risk.

(9) *Dietary factors*. Apart from constituents of the diet which may directly influence blood lipid levels, several others have been proposed as important in coronary heart disease risk. These include total energy intake, dietary fibre, salt, alcohol, and drinking water (degree of hardness).

Dietary factors in coronary heart disease

Total energy intake. A low intake of total energy has been associated with a high incidence of coronary heart disease; it is possible that the low energy intake is a consequence of a low energy output and a sedentary life style. Thus low levels of physical activity may explain the relationship.

Dietary fibre. A high intake of cereal fibre has been associated with a low incidence of coronary heart disease. It has been suggested that there may be an effect on plasma fibrinogen levels, and therefore reductions in the blood clotting tendency and consequent thrombosis.

Fruit and vegetable fibre, which contains viscous materials such as pectin, is reported as having cholesterol-lowering effects and may therefore also be of benefit, but via a different mechanism.

Salt. The supposed links between salt intake and raised blood pressure (hypertension) have been described in Chapter 7. Since hypertension is a recognized risk factor in coronary heart disease, it can be argued that reducing salt intake in those who are susceptible might reduce their coronary heart disease risk.

Alcohol. Heavy drinking is associated with considerable elevation of blood lipid levels and is therefore recognized as a risk factor in coronary heart disease. Other studies have suggested that a moderate alcohol intake may play a protective role, by increasing levels of the high density lipoproteins (HDL), which are believed to be beneficial. Interestingly, coronary heart disease mortality is greater at both ends of the range of alcohol consumption, in complete abstainers and in heavy drinkers, with a lower rate between these consumption levels.

Hardness of water. Total coronary heart disease mortality has been found to be lower in regions where the drinking water is hard, compared with soft-water areas. Of the minerals present in hard water, calcium and magnesium have been most studied. However, no conclusive theory about their protective effects has yet been constructed.

From this brief review of the risk factors involved in coronary heart disease, it should be clear that a great number of interactions are possible.

Blood lipid levels

Much attention has been focussed on attempts to reduce coronary heart disease by manipulating the blood lipid levels. Much of the literature is devoted to the question of modifying blood lipids by diet.

Blood cholesterol. Blood cholesterol levels were originally the main focus of attention, as the fatty deposits in blood vessels were observed to consist primarily of cholesterol, albeit with other components like fibrin, calcium and blood cell fragments. In addition, the risk of heart disease in a population increases with increasing blood cholesterol levels.

Up to a point, blood cholesterol levels can be influenced by dietary intake of cholesterol; it must be remembered, however, that cholesterol is also synthesized by the liver, and that the absolute level in the blood is determined more by genetic make-up than by dietary cholesterol intake, which probably contributes only about 10%. As cholesterol intake increases, its absorption decreases; the response is probably not linear, so that very high intakes may cause elevations of blood cholesterol levels. Individual handling of dietary cholesterol is, however, very variable.

In addition, it was found that intakes of saturated fatty acids could raise the blood cholesterol level, whereas polyunsaturated fats could reduce it. The effect of the saturated fats in raising levels is more powerful than that of the polyunsaturated fats in lowering them.

Lipoproteins. With improvements in analytical techniques, it became possible to separate the blood lipids into their constituent fractions by density – the lipoproteins. Each of the major lipoproteins has specific functions, described fully in Chapter 5. The low density lipoproteins (LDL), as the major transport mechanism for cholesterol, have been recognized as the fraction most likely to be associated with coronary heart disease. HDL, conversely, have emerged as the protective fraction, as these appear to remove cholesterol from tissues and artery walls.

The mechanisms by which dietary fats influence lipoprotein fractions are not yet clearly understood.

Attention is now being turned to the ratio of cholesterol to HDL cholesterol as a more sensitive indicator of possible risk. Reductions in this ratio appear to be of benefit, with a ratio of 3.5 to 4.5 being desirable.

Essential fatty acids. A rather different view of the possible advantages of polyunsaturated fatty acids (PUFA) relates to the role of some of them as essential fatty acids. Diets high in saturated fats and low in PUFA may induce a deficiency of essential fatty acids. A significantly lower content of linoleic acid has been found in the adipose tissue of people dying from coronary heart disease in various countries, compared with controls.

Trans-fatty acids, found in some soft margarines which have been hydrogenated during processing, may increase the body's needs for linoleic acid and thus aggravate the deficiency.

Evidence is accumulating that oils in fatty fish may be beneficial in thrombosis. Initial observations on Greenland Eskimos demonstrated low blood clotting tendency. The diet is rich in very long-chain polyunsaturated fatty acids (especially eicosapentaenoic acid, 20:5), which are antithrombogenic, and may explain the very low incidence of heart disease in this population, despite a high fat intake. Some studies in the West have now started to include advice on increasing consumption of fatty fish, as a means of reducing heart disease risk.

Prevention trials

In order to test the involvement of some of the risk factors described above, a large number of studies have been carried out around the world. These have been both primary and secondary prevention studies, i.e. either attempting to reduce the occurrence of an initial heart attack, or preventing a recurrence.

Many of these studies have attempted to change several risk factors; as a result, their findings may be difficult to interpret. Some of the major studies are summarized in Table 17.1.

The results of these studies cannot provide firm proof that alteration in dietary fats is the major contributor to coronary heart disease reduction. In all of the studies listed, other factors have also been altered; the contribution of each to the overall change is unknown, or at best difficult to quantify. In addition problems have arisen with control groups, which have also improved their health practices, as a result of improved public health awareness. Some concern has arisen recently that excessive lowering of blood cholesterol may result in an increased cancer risk.

Many unanswered questions remain on the issue of diet and coronary heart disease. The rôle of dietary fats as contributors to altered plasma lipid level has gradually become clearer. Nevertheless the 'best' dietary fat mixture is still not

Table 17.1 Summary of some coronary heart disease prevention trials.

Name of study	Major advice/dietary change	Results
Finnish Mental Hospital Study (1979)	Reduce saturated fat Increase polyunsaturated fat	Fall in serum cholesterol; fall in cardiovascular deaths
Oslo Study (1981)	Reduce saturated fat Increase polyunsaturated fat Reduce energy in obese Stop smoking	Reduced cholesterol and triglyceride levels; major fall in heart disease mortality
Multiple Risk Factor Intervention Trial (MRFIT), USA (1982)	Reduce blood lipids by diet Reduce obesity Reduce blood pressure Stop smoking Increase activity	Both the study group and controls improved heart disease risk
Lipid Research Clinics (1984)	Cholesterol reduction by diet and by drugs	Major fall in heart disease mortality

Table 17.2 COMA recommendations for dietary change.

Food/nutrient	Recommendation
Total fat	35% of total energy
Saturated fatty acids	15% of total energy
Polyunsaturated fatty acids	6.8% of energy
P/S ratio (Polyunsaturated/saturated fat)	0.45
Cholesterol	No specific recommendation
Simple sugars	No further increase
Alcohol	Excessive intake avoided
Salt	No further increase; consider ways of decreasing it
Fibre-rich carbohydrates	Increase intake

(Note that these are intended for the general public. However, the recommendations on fat intakes are not intended for infants, or for children below the age of five who usually obtain a substantial proportion of dietary energy from cow's milk.) From: Committee on Medical Aspects of Food Policy (1984) *Report on the Prevention of Coronary Heart Disease*. London: HMSO.

known, with possible dangers in excessive intakes of polyunsaturated fatty acids, *trans*-fatty acids, saturated fats, or inadequate cholesterol levels.

There are also possible relationships between dietary fibre and coronary heart disease. The influence of diet on the blood clotting mechanisms is also being explored. Although much still remains to be clarified, the advice of bodies such as NACNE and COMA is based on current knowledge and suggests moderation in any dietary changes. The advice from COMA is summarized in Table 17.2.

In 1985, the National Institutes of Health Conference recommended intensive dietary intervention for all people in the USA in the top quarter of distribution of blood cholesterol values, with the use of drugs for the top 10% if dietary effects were inadequate. Applying these criteria in Britain would encompass half of all middle-aged men. The NIH recommendations were:

(1) Reduce total fat from 40% to 30% of total energy.
(2) Reduce saturated fat to less than 20% of total energy.
(3) Increase polyunsaturated fat to no more than 10% of total energy.

In general, policies should aim for an overall improvement in dietary pattern, with more resources aimed at the high-risk groups, but not to the exclusion of the wider population.

Dietary fibre and health

For much of this century, the role of dietary fibre in health has largely been ignored. The earliest editions of this book gave it only a passing mention. In the early 1970s, interest was awakened by reports that the low prevalence in rural Africa and Asia of intestinal diseases, common in the West, could be associated with the low intakes of dietary fibre in western countries. Further, diverticular disease of the colon, generally treated with a low-fibre diet, was found to improve greatly when a diet rich in dietary fibre was given. Evidence was also presented that dietary fibre might reduce the risk of other 'western diseases', such as coronary heart disease, diabetes and common bowel disorders.

A fibre hypothesis has been developed, which broadly states that:

(1) A diet rich in foods containing plant cell-wall material (i.e. unrefined plant foods, including cereals, vegetables and fruits) is protective against 'western diseases'.

(2) A diet which is depleted of such materials may in some cases cause 'western diseases', or in others be a factor facilitating their development.

The term 'dietary fibre' is misleadingly simple. It implies a single entity, with consistent and predictable properties. In reality, dietary fibre is a collective term for a number of diverse substances (described in Chapter 4), all having their origin in plants, but having differing physiological and chemical properties, and probably having varying effects in the body. As a result, general statements about 'the effects of dietary fibre on health' may not apply to some of the constituents of the fibre complex.

Before considering the relationship with health and disease, it is useful to review the physiological effects of fibre as it passes through the alimentary tract, from mouth to the anus. This is summarized in Table 17.3.

Table 17.3 Summary of the effects of dietary fibre on the gastro-intestinal tract.

	Effect of dietary fibre
Mouth	Increased chewing Increased saliva flow Better dental health
Stomach	Increased volume of contents Increased viscosity; slower emptying ? Poorer access of enzymes to food
Small intestine	Increased viscosity Slower digestion and absorption

Large intestine	Faster transit
	Increased bulk:
	    water retention
	    gas production
	    bacterial growth
	Dilution of contents
	Nutrient/waste product binding

Relationship of physiological effects to prevention of disease

Diseases that have been linked with an inadequate intake of dietary fibre, or may be relieved with an increased intake of fibre, may be grouped according to the major mechanisms believed to be involved. These are shown in Table 17.4. It must be remembered that some of the effects may overlap between groups.

Mechanical effects

Constipation. This is described as the difficult passage of small, hard stools. It appears to be particularly common in the West, although prevalence data are

Table 17.4 Relationship between fibre action and disease.

Nature of effect	Major condition/disease involved
Mechanical	Constipation
	Irritable bowel syndrome
	? Appendicitis
	Diverticular disease
	Haemorrhoids
	Hiatus hernia
Dilution	Obesity
	Dental disease
Absorption and adsorption	Diabetes
	Gallstones
	Coronary heart disease
	Cancer of the colon

scanty. Average stool weights in Britain are about 100 to 120 g per day (although 225 g in vegetarians). In Northern India, they are reported to be 310 g and approximately 500 g in rural Kenyans and Ugandans. This is attributed to the varying amounts of dietary fibre consumed. Low intakes of dietary fibre contribute to low stool weight; inclusion of wheat bran, preferably in the form of the whole cereal, increases stool bulk and relieves constipation. Fruit and vegetable fibre, high in pectins and fermentable fibre sources, has a less predictable effect on stool weight.

Irritable bowel syndrome. This generally presents as alternating diarrhoea and constipation, sometimes accompanied by pain. It is believed to be the result of an inappropriate reaction of the gut muscles to stress and physical conditions in the gut. Lack of dietary fibre may be one of the precipitating factors. Increasing the intake of cereal fibre alleviates the symptoms in a proportion of patients.

Appendicitis. The incidence of appendicitis is linked with economic development and affluence, even within individuals from the same ethnic group. It has been suggested that obstruction of the appendix with hard faecaliths is more likely on a low-fibre diet with damage to the mucosal lining. However, this is probably not the cause in all cases of appendicitis.

Diverticular disease. Diverticulae are 'blow-outs' of the mucosa of the colon, producing blind pockets within the wall. These may become inflamed (diverticulitis) or even perforated; both of these cause pain. Diverticulae are believed to be present within the colon in 50 to 70% of the over-80s in the West.

They are believed to develop as follows: when the colon contents are small and dry, high pressure must be generated by the colonic muscles to propel the contents along. The muscles hypertrophy, or thicken over a period of time. The colon becomes highly segmented, generating very high pressures locally which weaken the mucosa, eventually resulting in a 'blow-out'.

In the early 1970s, bran was used to relieve the symptoms, with considerable success. Coarse wheat bran is more effective than fine bran because of its great water-holding capacity. Whole cereals are now recommended. Vegetarians rarely develop diverticular disease, suggesting a role for dietary fibre in prevention.

Haemorrhoids. This term refers to the downward displacement of the specialized submucosal anal cushions into the opening of the anus. They may bleed and cause discomfort. Hard stools are likely to damage their surface, and possibly cause further displacement. Softer stools will not cause such damage. A high-fibre diet has been shown to provide relief.

Hiatus hernia. The displacement of the upper part of the stomach through the diaphragm is known as hiatus hernia. There is an increased tendency for stomach contents to reflux into the lower oesophagus, causing pain (heartburn). Hiatus hernia has a prevalence of 1% in developing countries, and 10 to 35% in the West. It has been postulated that straining to evacuate small, hard faeces causes increased upward pressure on the stomach, causing it to herniate through the diaphragm. However, this theory is not supported by experimental study.

Dilution effects

Dental disease. The prevalence of dental caries is low in those who eat an unrefined and unprocessed diet; this is reversed when refined foods are added. These groups also have a low incidence of periodontal disease. The role of dietary fibre in dental disease has been described in Chapter 16, and is summarized here:

(1) High-fibre foods require more chewing and therefore stimulate salivary flow.

(2) Saliva helps to remove food debris from teeth and buffers any acids produced.

(3) Water-soluble substances, probably phosphates present in fibre-rich foods, may have a remineralizing effect.

(4) Regular chewing of hard foods hardens the gums and may flatten and smooth tooth surfaces, reducing potential sites for plaque accumulation.

Obesity. In the early 1980s a book entitled *The F-Plan Diet* was a major best-seller in the UK. Its main message was the consumption of a diet containing up to 40 g of dietary fibre and low in energy content. The theme was that this would result in weight loss without hunger.

Low dietary fibre intakes may play a part in the development of obesity in several ways:

(1) Fibre-depleted foods, especially those containing sugars, produce very short-term satiety. They are also energy-rich and highly palatable, leading to over-consumption.

(2) Fibre-rich foods provide satiety, reduce the concentration of energy in foods, slow nutrient absorption and prevent large fluctuations in blood glucose level, which may be a cause of hunger.

Absorption and adsorption

Diabetes mellitus. Maturity onset or non-insulin-dependent diabetes is frequently associated with overweight. Rapid absorption of nutrients – particularly glucose – from the small intestine causes a large insulin response. This in turn lowers the blood glucose level, sometimes below 'normal' levels: this is called 'rebound hypoglycaemia'. Such extreme swings of blood glucose level are undesirable, both in the normal individual and particularly in diabetics.

Consuming a high-fibre diet reduces the blood glucose peak seen after meals. Thus normal individuals can benefit as well as diabetics, in whom better control can be obtained and insulin dosages reduced.

The high-fibre diet can be useful both in the prevention and treatment of diabetes. A further advantage is that a high-fibre diet can contain less fat, thus possibly reducing complications such as heart disease, as well as the incidence of obesity in the diabetic. The most effective dietary fibre sources for diabetics are pectins, legume fibre and guar gum, all of which increase viscosity in the gut and slow absorption. However, cereal fibre can also be of benefit in improving blood glucose control and blood triglyceride levels.

Gallstones. In the West, gallstones are composed predominantly of cholesterol; the other major components are calcium salts. Gallstones are thought to be produced when the bile in the gallbladder becomes supersaturated with cholesterol and precipitates out into crystals, forming stones. Supersaturation arises from excessive levels of cholesterol, insufficient bile salts to maintain the cholesterol in suspension, or both of these.

As the incidence of gallstones is greater in the West and rare in developing countries, links with dietary fibre are proposed. The suggested mechanism for dietary fibre in protecting against gallstones is shown in Fig. 17.1.

The mucilaginous and gel-forming polysaccharides (e.g. pectin) and lignin are most effective in bile acid binding.

Coronary heart disease. Coronary heart disease has been shown to be less common in individuals with high intakes of dietary fibre than in those with low intake levels. Inverse relationships with both total fibre and cereal fibre intakes have been found. Vegetable fibre sources may cause increased cholesterol excretion, via bile acids. Cereal fibre does not affect cholesterol levels, but may influence blood clotting mechanisms.

Large bowel (colon) cancer. Colon cancer is the most common fatal cancer in the USA and the second most common in the UK. Several theories have been proposed for the twenty-fold variation in incidence of colon cancer throughout the world. Migrants tend towards the colon cancer rate of their adopted country, suggesting an environmental influence. Significant negative associations have

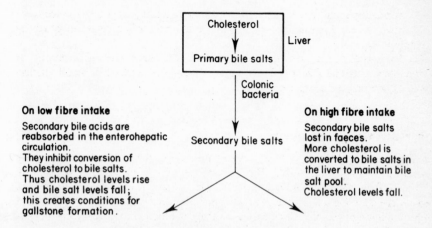

Fig. 17.1 Suggested role of dietary fibre in bile acid excretion and cholesterol metabolism.

been shown between colon cancer occurrence and dietary fibre intakes in Scandinavia and Britain. The intake of pentoses gives the best negative correlation with colon cancer rates.

Several mechanisms have been proposed:

(1) The concentration of any carcinogen in the stools will be lower in bulky, dilute stools than in hard, dry ones.

(2) Slow transit of a fibre-depleted diet will prolong the exposure time of the colon to harmful substances.

(3) Ammonia is produced in the colon by microbial action of nitrogen-waste products. This may be excreted in the faeces or taken up by bacteria. Bacterial growth, stimulated by fibre, will take up the ammonia, reducing faecal ammonia content and any harm this might cause.

(4) A high-fibre diet causes a low faecal pH, due to the volatile fatty acids produced by the bacteria. These include butyric acid which is an important substrate for energy metabolism by the colon cells. A low pH also reduces bile acid breakdown and ammonia uptake by cells.

Although the exact mechanisms for the development of colonic cancer are unknown, the protective role of dietary fibre, indicated by epidemiology, may thus operate through several routes.

Excessive intakes of dietary fibre

Although the foregoing discussion suggests that dietary fibre is beneficial for health, it is necessary to practise some caution in its intake.

(1) A sudden switch to a high-fibre diet can cause abdominal distension and pain, with possible diarrhoea. Thus intakes of dietary fibre should be increased gradually.

(2) Occasionally, an obstruction may arise, particularly where there is some pre-existing abnormality in the gut.

(3) High-fibre diets tend to increase faecal loss of minerals, so that people who have marginally adequate intakes may become deficient. This is particularly important in Asians in the UK, where a high-fibre diet is believed to contribute to the incidence of poor bone status.

In addition, the presence of phytic acid in a whole-cereal diet may further reduce the availability of minerals for absorption.

Low iron, zinc or calcium intakes may become too low if fibre is increased excessively. In particular the use of bran is to be discouraged, as this binds many minerals. Natural, whole sources of dietary fibre, like fruit, vegetables and whole-grain cereal foods provide additional minerals, which can offset the reduced absorption.

(4) People with small appetites require food with a high nutrient density; fibre-rich foods dilute the diet. As a result, the increased volume cannot be eaten and an inadequate intake results. Thus it is important not to give too much fibre to young children, elderly people and the sick. In all cases, some fibre is needed, but only in addition to other nutrients, rather than in their place (as might occur with bran).

Table 17.5 Cancers and their possible nutrition links.

Cancer site	Possible nutrition link(s)
Oesophagus	Excess alcohol
Stomach	Salt Nitrosamines ? Green vegetables protective (? vitamin C)
Liver	Excess alcohol
Colon/rectum	Large fat intake Large meat intake Dietary fibre protective
Lung	Vitamin A protective
Breast/uterus	Overweight Large fat intake Dietary fibre protective
Bladder	Vitamin A protective Nitrosamines Coffee
Prostate	Large fat intake

Nutrition and cancer

It has been claimed that about 50% of cancers in the USA and the UK could be diet-related. Since cancer is a major cause of morbidity and death, it is important that these dietary factors are studied in an attempt to improve public health. However, at present no conclusive proof exists that changing a specific element in the diet will have an important effect on cancer incidence.

The ways in which food or nutrients may contribute to the development of cancer may be broadly classified as follows:

(1) Foods may be a source of preformed (or precursors of) carcinogens.
(2) Nutrients may affect the formation, transport, deactivation and excretion of carcinogens.
(3) Nutrients may affect the resistance of the body's cells to carcinogens.

Some of the sites in the body where a nutritional link with cancer has been proposed are summarized in Table 17.5.

The same nutritional links appear in several of the specific cancers listed in Table 17.5, and therefore appear at present to be the more likely causative/preventive agents.

Overweight and total energy intake

Restricting the food intake in mice, without modifying the proportion of its individual nutrients, has long been known to halve the incidence of spontaneous tumours of the breast and lung, and reduce susceptibility to known carcinogens.

A major 13-year study of 750 000 Americans has largely confirmed this finding in humans.

For women, there is a consistent trend towards increasing total cancer risk, particularly that of the womb, with increasing body weight. In men the trend is less clear, as lung cancer – which is linked with low body weight – is more dominant.

A smaller trend to higher incidence in the overweight for cancers of the gall-bladder, cervix, ovary, colon/rectum and breast was also reported.

High fat intake

An association in populations, but not so strongly in individuals, has been shown between the intake of fat and the occurrence of cancer of the colon, breast, endometrium (womb), ovary and prostate. All of these show geographical associations. Apart from colon cancer, the remainder appear to be hormone-related.

In the case of colon cancer, it is known that a higher fat intake results in a greater excretion of bile acids in the faeces. Under the anaerobic conditions present in the intestines, bile acids are metabolized to mutagenic compounds.

In some populations, the relationship between fat and colon cancer does not hold. Other dietary factors are likely to play a modifying role. The foremost of these is dietary fibre. A relationship has been proposed with vegetable intake, which may play a protective role through its vitamin C content, or the presence of indoles. Finally, vitamin E may abolish the mutagenic activity in the faeces.

The correlation with fat and hormone-linked cancers has been studied particularly for breast and endometrial cancer. A high fat intake causes an excessive endogenous production of oestrogens from cholesterol metabolites in the gut. In addition oestrogen levels are linked to adiposity. Breast cancers in postmenopausal women tend to be oestrogen-dependent, and may thus respond to these raised hormone levels. In addition breast cancer is linked with early menarche and late menopause, both of which are related to a high plane of nutrition in early life and obesity.

However, it has been recently suggested that a deficit in dietary fibre can reduce oestrogen levels, and therefore delay menarche and uterine development. The negative correlation of breast and endometrial cancers with dietary fibre is reportedly stronger than their positive association with fat.

Finally, there is a possibility that low blood cholesterol levels increase the risk of colon cancer, particularly in males.

Dietary fibre

The role of dietary fibre in the colon, particularly in relation to colon cancer, has been discussed earlier in this chapter. In particular, pentosans (from whole cereals) and vegetables (but not potatoes) show negative correlations with colon cancer death rates.

Vitamin A

Animal studies have shown that vitamin A delays the development of cancer, and a deficiency of the vitamin enhances the susceptibility of animals to cancer. Vitamin A consists of two distinct groups of substances – retinoids and carotenoids – which must be considered separately.

Foods of animal origin supply vitamin A as retinol, which is transported around the body attached to retinol binding protein. The blood concentrations of carrier-bound retinol are largely independent of liver retinol stores and dietary intake, and cannot therefore be raised by increasing retinol intakes. However, studies in Norway and London have found twice the incidence of cancer among subjects whose plasma retinol levels were lower than controls. How to raise blood retinol levels remains a mystery, however.

The chief carotenoid present in the diet is beta-carotene, which is mostly converted to retinal and retinol during absorption. Some, however, is absorbed unchanged, and blood and tissue levels are directly related to intakes over the previous weeks. In Japan, it has been shown that the incidence of cancer was lower by half in those people who ate green or yellow vegetables daily compared with controls. Also, a 19-year study in the USA of middle-aged men found an inverse relationship between carotene intake and lung cancer.

Retinoids regulate cell differentiation and could therefore influence tumour growth. Carotenoids are extremely efficient at inactivating 'excited oxygen', protecting cells from damage.

Two other nutrients which might play a similar role in protecting cells against oxidative damage are vitamin E and selenium. There are some studies indicating a higher incidence of cancers (especially of the alimentary tract) in areas where selenium levels are low, and in people consuming low vitamin E intakes. In both cases, more information is needed.

Salt

The occurrence of stomach cancer has been linked with a number of nutritional factors. These include nitrates or nitrites, salty, pickled or smoked foods, vitamin C and fresh fruit and vegetables. Mortality from stomach cancer has been decreasing around the world for several decades. Until recently, no apparent link with any specific nutritional factors could be identified. However, it was noted that gastric cancer mortality was strongly related to stroke mortality. This was true between countries, between different regions of the same country, and different subgroups of the population. The relationship is so strong that a linking factor is implicated. It has been suggested that this factor is salt.

Salt has a high osmotic activity and has been reported to cause gastritis in animals.

The decline in stroke mortality and gastric cancer may be explained by decreases in salt intake with advances in food preservation. Refrigeration and deep freezing have reduced the use of salt as a preservative for meat, fish and vegetables. However, there is still a higher salt intake in lower socio-economic groups, reflected in their higher rate of stomach cancer.

It is likely that salt is still a major (but possibly not the only) nutritional cause of stomach cancer.

Nitrosamines

Nitrosamines are produced in the body by the reaction of nitrites with secondary and tertiary amines. Nitrites originate both by bacterial action on dietary nitrate and from addition to food as preservatives. Vegetables are particularly rich in nitrates; drinking water may be another source. Nitrosable compounds are derived

Table 17.6 Dietary guidelines for the prevention of cancer.

Food/nutrient	Advice
Saturated and unsaturated fats	Reduce to 30% of total energy
Additional vitamins: A, C and E and dietary fibre	From inclusion of fruit, vegetable and wholegrain cereal products. Use of potentially toxic nutrient supplements is discouraged
Salt-cured or smoked foods	Minimize intake
Carcinogenic substances in foods	Avoid, or keep to permissible levels
Alcohol	In moderation

predominantly from meat and fish; formation of nitrosamines could in theory occur with a number of normal dietary combinations. It is enhanced by thiocyanate ions (from tobacco smoke) and inhibited by antioxidants (e.g. vitamin C) in the stomach.

Although nitrosamines have been shown to be carcinogenic in animal tissues, there is little evidence that the oesophageal and gastric cancers found in some parts of the world can be attributed to nitrosamines. Indeed, there appears to be an inverse relationship between vegetable intake and gastric cancer, suggesting that these nitrates are not contributing to the risk. An explanation may be the presence in vegetables of vitamin C, which inhibits nitrosamine formation.

Dietary guidelines for the prevention of cancer were formulated in 1982 by a committee of the American National Academy of Sciences. They are based on evidence such as that described above. Although it is not yet possible to be certain about some of the associations between diet and cancer, the committee felt that the evidence was sufficiently convincing to propose interim dietary guidelines. These are summarized in Table 17.6.

The committee emphasized that the cooperation of the health professions and food industry would be required to implement the guidelines.

Obesity

Obesity is a serious and frequent health hazard in affluent societies. Medical complications found in the obese include diabetes, hypertension, gallstones, raised blood lipids and disease of the womb in women. Obesity can increase the risk of many of the conditions already discussed in this chapter.

Obesity arises from an imbalance of energy intake over energy output. The daily discrepancy need not be very great for a steady increase in weight to occur. The relative contribution of factors to the imbalance has been the subject of much investigation.

Childhood obesity

Overweight in childhood does not necessarily result in adult overweight. A study in Britain of the weights of people as children, and as adults, found that less than half of the overweight 7-year-olds became overweight adults. Similar evidence comes from a study in New York, with 36% of overweight infants being overweight 20 to 30 years later; the figure for average weight infants was 14%.

Genetic influence

The extent of genetic influence is difficult to separate from that of the environment. However, studies on identical and non-identical twins raised separately or together, and on adopted children and their natural and adopting parents, suggest that genetic influences do contribute to overweight. A figure of approximately 50% of body fat being determined by inheritance has been proposed. A recent (1986) study in Denmark found very high correlations for body mass index with natural parents, and no relationship with those of adoptive parents.

Metabolic factors

Hormonal abnormalities are very rarely a cause of overweight, although they may result from overweight. The most important example of the latter is diabetes mellitus of the non-insulin-dependent type, which is very frequently associated with overweight. In addition, menstrual and reproductive difficulties may arise in overweight women.

The metabolic basis of overweight has been much studied. The BMR of obese individuals is higher than those of normal weight, as explained in Chapter 3. It was suggested in the early 1980s that there was a poorer ability in obese people to generate heat in their brown adipose tissue, in response to overeating. The brown adipose tissue in animals has been demonstrated to be a site of heat production, which hypertrophies on excessive food intake. The intake of carbohydrates in particular is believed to stimulate it. From this it was postulated that a similar mechanism might operate in humans, with lean individuals having particularly effective brown fat, whereas that of the obese was in some way defective. Measurements of metabolic rate in response to eating have not provided conclusive evidence.

Nevertheless, the results of many studies do suggest that there is a metabolic difference between people in their ability to waste food energy, so that overfeeding does not result in the same degree of weight gain in everyone.

If lower metabolism cannot fully explain weight gain, the answer may lie in higher energy intakes. Careful measurements of normal food intakes have suggested that the overweight do eat more than they actually admit to eating, suggesting that this may be a contributory factor.

Physical activity

Physical activity involves an increase in energy expenditure and is therefore likely to limit weight gain. The effects of physical exercise in relation to total energy turnover each day may be small, but these small differences may add up to affect energy balance.

There has been a gradual decline in physical activity of the population as a whole, which has probably contributed to the increase in overweight. The NACNE report, in recognizing this, made strong recommendations that exercise should be maintained throughout life and not just in schoolchildren and young adults. Thus an increase in exercise for the whole community is needed, with better facilities; overweight individuals in particular should be encouraged to be more active.

Social aspects

Obesity carries a social stigma in certain sections of affluent societies. On the other hand, there is continued pressure to eat. This conflict can make people confused, so that food intake becomes disordered. For example, pressure to eat comes from parents, the food industry, advertizing and the variety of foods available. There are also social pressures, which include those related to social class and gender. The drinking of alcohol can also contribute to excessive energy intake.

Energy output may also be subject to social pressure; it has traditionally been less acceptable for women to engage in sport, although this is now changing.

Psychological aspects

It has been suggested that individuals overeat and become obese for psychological reasons. This is compared to other forms of stress-induced behaviour, such as smoking or nail-biting. Indeed, carbohydrate addiction has been proposed, with the addict craving carbohydrate in the way that others crave alcohol, drugs or cigarettes.

Treatment of obesity

Many ways of treating obesity and overweight have been used. Their common objective is to reduce the amount of energy taken as food and/or to increase the amount of energy expended by the body. Ideally, weight loss should be slow (0.5 kg per week) and steady, and at the same time dietary and activity habits should be re-educated. Treatments include:

(1) Weight-reducing diets – supervised or unsupervised. These may include eating less normal food, or a special 'calorie counted food', or concentrating on particular components of the diet (high fibre, low fat, low carbohydrate, high protein, etc.).
(2) Use of appetite suppressants.
(3) Behaviour therapy.
(4) Surgical intervention:
  jaw wiring
  intestinal bypass
  stapling of stomach
  intragastric balloons.
(5) Starvation therapy.
(6) Exercise.

In terms of public health, prevention of obesity is better than cure. The NACNE report made several recommendations for maintenance of body weight, based on the Royal College of Physicians report on obesity in 1983. These recommendations are summarized as follows:

(1) The prevention of weight gain is important, particularly in those with a familial pattern of diabetes, hypertension and heart disease.

(2) Weight gain on stopping smoking should be prevented by adjustment of the diet.

(3) Overweight in children should be avoided, particularly by reducing intakes of dietary fats and sugars. Fibre-rich starchy foods should not be reduced.

(4) Improved food labelling with respect to fat, sugar and energy contents would be of benefit.

(5) Physical activity should be maintained for life.

(6) Diets for weight reduction should include plenty of cereals, bread, fruit and vegetables, and restrict foods rich in fats and sugars. Behaviour modification is helpful for long-term alteration of life style.

References and Further Reading

General

Birch, G.G., Cameron, A.G., Spencer, M. (1986). *Food Science*. Oxford: Pergamon Press.
Department of Health and Social Security (1979). *Recommended Daily Amounts of Food Energy and Nutrients for Groups of People in the United Kingdom (Report 15)*. London: HMSO.
Passmore, R., Eastwood, M.A. (1986). *Davidson and Passmore: Human Nutrition and Dietetics*. Edinburgh: Churchill Livingstone.
Paul, A.A., Southgate, D.A.T. (1978). *McCance and Widdowson's The Composition of Foods*. London: HMSO.

The Lancet, New Scientist and *Scientific American* are recommended reading for up-to-date information.

Chapter 1

British Nutrition Foundation (1985). *Eating in the Early 1980s; Attitudes and Behaviour*. London: BNF.
Medical Research Council Environmental Epidemiology Unit (1984). *The Dietary Assessment of Populations* (Science Report 4). London: MRC.
Wright, R.A., Heymsfield. S., McManus, C.B. (1984). *Nutritional Assessment*. Oxford: Blackwell Scientific Publications.

Chapter 2

National Advisory Committee on Nutrition Education (1983). *Proposals for Nutritional Guidelines for Health Education in Britain*. London: Health Education Council.
Tan, S.P., Wenlock, R.W.; Buss, D.H. (1985). *Immigrant Foods* (Second Supplement to McCance and Widdowson's *The Composition of Foods*). London: HMSO.
United States Department of Agriculture (1976–1985). *Composition of Foods Raw, Processed and Prepared*. (Agriculture Handbook No. 8, parts 1–13). Washington: USDA.

Chapter 3

Garrow, J.S. (1981). *Treat Obesity Seriously*. Edinburgh: Churchill Livingstone.

Chapter 9

Committee on Dietary Allowances, Food and Nutrition Board (1980). *Recommended Dietary Allowances*, 9th edn. Washington: National Academy of Sciences.
FAO/WHO/UNU Expert Consultation (1985). *Energy and Protein Requirements*. Geneva: WHO.

Chapter 10

Committee on Medical Aspects of Food Policy, Department of Health and Social Security (1984). *Diet and Cardiovascular Disease.* London: HMSO.
Department of Health and Social Security (1981). *Nutritional Aspects of Bread and Flour.* London: HMSO.
National Food Survey Committee annual reports. *Household Food Consumption and Expenditure.* London: HMSO.

Chapter 11

The British Dietetic Association (1985). *The Great British Diet.* London: Century Hutchinson.
Maryon-Davis, A., Thomas, J. (1984). *Diet 2000: How to eat for a healthier future.* London: Pan.

Chapter 12

Lennon, D. and Fieldhouse, P. (1982) *Social Nutrition.* London: Forbes Publications.
Turner, M. (Ed.) (1980). *Nutrition and Lifestyles.* London: Applied Science Publishers.

Chapter 13

Abraham, S., and Llewellyn-Jones, D. (1984). *Eating Disorders – The Facts.* Oxford: Oxford Medical Publications.
Bull, N.L. (1986). *Dietary habits of 15–25 year olds.* In *Human Nutrition; Applied Nutrition Supplement.* London: John Libbey.
Davies, L. (1982). *Three Score Years . . . And Then?* London: Heinemann.
Department of Health and Social Security (1979). *Nutrition and Health in Old Age (Report 16).* London: HMSO.
Department of Health and Social Security (1980). *Artificial Feeds for the Young Infant (Report 18).* London: HMSO.
Francis, D. (1986). *Nutrition for Children.* Oxford: Blackwell Scientific Publications.
Hunt, J. (1986). *A Vegetarian in the Family.* Wellingborough: Thorsons.
National Dairy Council (1981). *What are children eating these days?* London: NDC.
Wenlock, R.W., Disselduff, M.M., Skinner R.K., Knight, I. (1986). *Diets of British Schoolchildren.* London: HMSO.

Chapter 14

Asians in Britain (1976). Burgess Hill: Van den Berghs & Jurgens Ltd.
Berry Ottaway, P., Hargin, K. (1985). *Food for Sport: A handbook of sports nutrition.* Resource Publications.
Campbell, D.M., Gillmer, M.D.G. (eds) (1982). *Nutrition in Pregnancy.* London: Royal College of Obstetricians and Gynaecologists.
Cole-Hamilton, I. and Lang, T. (1986) *Tightening Belts – A report on the impact of poverty on food.* London: Food Commission.
Townsend, P. and Davidson, N. (eds) (1982). *Inequalities in Health: The Black Report.* London: Penguin Books.

Chapter 15

Eagle, R. (1986). *Eating and Allergy.* Wellingborough: Thorsons.
Forbes, A. (1985). *The Bristol Diet.* London: Century Hutchinson.

Howard, A. (1985). *The Cambridge Diet*. London: Jonathan Cape.
Royal College of Physicians and British Nutrition Foundation (1984). *Food intolerance and food aversion*. London: RCP.

Chapter 16

Cook, R., Cook, E. (1983). *Sugar Off: The good tooth food guide*. Cambridge: Great Ouse Press.
Health Education Council (1985). *The Scientific Basis of Dental Health Education*. London: HEC.
Royal College of Physicians (1976). *Fluoride, teeth and health*. London: Pitman Medical.

Chapter 17

Eyton, A. (1982). *The F-Plan Diet*. London: Penguin.
National Academy of Sciences Committee on Diet, Nutrition and Cancer (1982). *Diet, Nutrition and Cancer*. Washington: National Academy Press.
Royal College of Physicians (1980) *Medical Aspects of Dietary Fibre*. London: Pitman Medical.
Royal College of Physicians (1983). *Obesity*. London: RCP.

Index

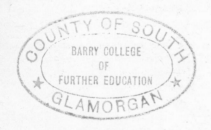